Deborah F. Glazer, PhD
Jack Drescher, MD
Editors

Gay and Lesbian Parenting

Gay and Lesbian Parenting has been co-published simultaneously as *Journal of Gay & Lesbian Psychotherapy*, Volume 4, Numbers 3/4 2001.

Pre-Publication
REVIEWS,
COMMENTARIES,
EVALUATIONS . . .

"**A** WELCOME AND AFFIRMING RESOURCE FOR GAY AND LESBIAN PERSONS AND THEIR THERAPISTS. . . . Offers readers many maps to explore the territory."

Maggie Magee
Diana C. Miller
authors of Lesbians Lives:
Psychoanalytic Narratives
Old and New

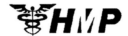

The Haworth Medical Press
An Imprint of The Haworth Press, Inc.

Gay and Lesbian Parenting

Gay and Lesbian Parenting has been co-published simultaneously as *Journal of Gay & Lesbian Psychotherapy,* Volume 4, Numbers 3/4 2001.

The *Journal of Gay & Lesbian Psychotherapy* Monographic "Separates"

Below is a list of "separates," which in serials librarianship means a special issue simultaneously published as a special journal issue or double-issue *and* as a "separate" hardbound monograph. (This is a format which we also call a "DocuSerial.")

"Separates" are published because specialized libraries or professionals may wish to purchase a specific thematic issue by itself in a format which can be separately cataloged and shelved, as opposed to purchasing the journal on an on-going basis. Faculty members may also more easily consider a "separate" for classroom adoption.

"Separates" are carefully classified separately with the major book jobbers so that the journal tie-in can be noted on new book order slips to avoid duplicate purchasing.

You may wish to visit Haworth's website at . . .

http://www.HaworthPress.com

. . . to search our online catalog for complete tables of contents of these separates and related publications.

You may also call 1-800-HAWORTH (outside US/Canada: 607-722-5857), or Fax: 1-800-895-0582 (outside US/Canada: 607-771-0012), or e-mail at:

getinfo@haworthpressinc.com

Gay and Lesbian Parenting, edited by Deborah F. Glazer, PhD, and Jack Drescher, MD (Vol. 4, No. 3/4, 2001). *Richly textured, probing. These papers establish a rare feat: they explore in a candid, psychologically sophisticated, yet highly readable fashion, how parenthood impacts lesbian and gay identity and how these identities affect the experience of parenting. Wonderfully informative. (Martin Stephen Frommer, PhD, Faculty/Supervisor, The Institute for Contemporary Psychotherapy, New York City)*

Addictions in the Gay and Lesbian Community, edited by Jeffrey R. Guss, MD, and Jack Drescher, MD (Vol. 3, No. 3/4, 2000). *Explores the unique clinical considerations involved in addiction treatment for gay men and lesbians, groups that reportedly use and abuse alcohol and substances at higher rates than the general population.*

Gay and Lesbian Parenting

Deborah F. Glazer, PhD
Jack Drescher, MD
Editors

Gay and Lesbian Parenting has been co-published simultaneously as *Journal of Gay & Lesbian Psychotherapy*, Volume 4, Numbers 3/4 2001.

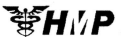

The Haworth Medical Press
An Imprint of
The Haworth Press, Inc.
New York • London • Oxford

Published by

The Haworth Medical Press®, 10 Alice Street, Binghamton, NY 13904-1580, USA

The Haworth Medical Press® is an imprint of The Haworth Press, Inc., 10 Alice Street, Binghamton, NY 13904-1580 USA.

Gay and Lesbian Parenting has been co-published simultaneously as *Journal of Gay & Lesbian Psychotherapy* ™, Volume 4, Numbers 3/4 2001.

The development, preparation, and publication of this work has been undertaken with great care. However, the publisher, employees, editors, and agents of The Haworth Press and all imprints of The Haworth Press, Inc., including The Haworth Medical Press® and Pharmaceutical Products Press®, are not responsible for any errors contained herein or for consequences that may ensue from use of materials or information contained in this work. Opinions expressed by the author(s) are not necessarily those of The Haworth Press, Inc.

Cover design by Jennifer Gaska

Library of Congress Cataloging-in-Publication Data

Gay and lesbian parenting / Deborah F. Glazer, Jack Drescher, editors.
     p. cm.
     "Co-published simultaneously as Journal of gay & lesbian psychotherapy, volume 4, numbers 3/4 2001."
     Includes bibliographical references and index.
     ISBN 0-7890-1349-5 (alk. paper) – ISBN 0-7890-1350-9 (alk. paper)
     1. Gay parents–United States. 2. Lesbian mothers–United States. 3. Children of gay parents–United States. 4. Parenting–United States. I. Glazer, Deborah F. II. Drescher, Jack, 1951- III. Journal of gay & lesbian psychotherapy.

HQ75.28.U6 G39 2001
306.874–dc21

2001039150

Indexing, Abstracting & Website/Internet Coverage

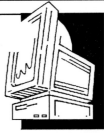

This section provides you with a list of major indexing & abstracting services. That is to say, each service began covering this periodical during the year noted in the right column. Most Websites which are listed below have indicated that they will either post, disseminate, compile, archive, cite or alert their own Website users with research-based content from this work. (This list is as current as the copyright date of this publication.)

Abstracting, Website/Indexing Coverage .... Year When Coverage Began

- *Abstracts in Anthropology* **1991**
- *Academic Index (on-line)* **1992**
- *Academic Search Elite (ERSCO)* **1998**
- *BUBL Information Service: An Internet-based Information
    Service for the UK higher education community
    <URL: http://bubl.ac.uk/>* **1995**
- *CNPIEC Reference Guide: Chinese National Directory
    of Foreign Periodicals* **1995**
- *Contemporary Women's Issues* **1998**
- *e-psyche, LLC <www.nisc.com>* **2001**
- *Expanded Academic ASAP <www.galegroup.com>* **1993**
- *Expanded Academic Index* **1995**
- *Family Studies Database (online and CD/ROM) <www.nisc.com>* **1998**
- *Family Violence & Sexual Assault Bulletin* **1992**
- *FINDEX <www.publist.com>* **1999**
- *Gay & Lesbian Abstracts <www.nisc.com>* **1999**
- *GenderWatch <www.slinfo.com>* **1999**
- *HOMODOK/"Relevant" Bibliographic database,
    Documentation Centre for Gay & Lesbian Studies,
    University of Amsterdam (selective printed abstracts
    in "Homologie" and bibliographic computer databases
    covering cultural, historical, social and political
    aspects of gay & lesbian topics)* **1995**

(continued)

Special Bibliographic Notes related to special journal issues (separates) and indexing/abstracting:

- indexing/abstracting services in this list will also cover material in any "separate" that is co-published simultaneously with Haworth's special thematic journal issue or DocuSerial. Indexing/abstracting usually covers material at the article/chapter level.
- monographic co-editions are intended for either non-subscribers or libraries which intend to purchase a second copy for their circulating collections.
- monographic co-editions are reported to all jobbers/wholesalers/approval plans. The source journal is listed as the "series" to assist the prevention of duplicate purchasing in the same manner utilized for books-in-series.
- to facilitate user/access services all indexing/abstracting services are encouraged to utilize the co-indexing entry note indicated at the bottom of the first page of each article/chapter/contribution.
- this is intended to assist a library user of any reference tool (whether print, electronic, online, or CD-ROM) to locate the monographic version if the library has purchased this version but not a subscription to the source journal.
- individual articles/chapters in any Haworth publication are also available through the Haworth Document Delivery Service (HDDS).

Gay and Lesbian Parenting

CONTENTS

ABOUT THE EDITORS

Deborah F. Glazer, PhD, is a faculty member and senior supervisor at the Psychoanalytic Institute of the Post-graduate Center for Mental Health and is on the faculty of the Institute for Human Identity and the Psychoanalytic Psychotherapy Study Center. Dr. Glazer serves on the editorial board of the *Journal of Gay & Lesbian Psychotherapy*. She is a psychologist/psychoanalyst in private practice in the Chelsea section of New York City.

Jack Drescher, MD, Editor-in-Chief of the *Journal of Gay & Lesbian Psychotherapy*, is Supervisor of Psychoanalysis and Faculty Member at the William Alanson White Psychoanalytic Institute and Clinical Assistant Professor of Psychiatry at the State University of New York-Brooklyn. Dr. Drescher chairs both the Committee on Gay, Lesbian and Bisexual Issues of the American Psychiatric Association and the Committee on Human Sexuality of the Group for the Advancement of Psychiatry. Author of *Psychoanalytic Therapy and the Gay Man* (1998, The Analytic Press), Dr. Drescher is in full-time private practice in New York City.

Introduction

At a party of two-mom families in a rural New York town, one mother turns to the other and asks "Which one of you gets up at night?" Both women laugh, as they reflect on their situations. They note that these are the mundane, daily issues that the "right" never discusses when they rail against homosexuality. At the same time, these are never the issues either woman expected to be dealing with when they came out 20 years ago.

This is the irony of gay and lesbian parenting. As April Martin notes later in this volume, gay and lesbian parenting is a "radical thing." It also seems that compiling this work is a "radical thing." Throughout the history of psychology and psychoanalysis, discussion of homosexuality has focused on questions of etiology and cure. Much work in the last decade has focused on depathologizing homosexuality while offering alternative developmental perspectives (Schwartz, 1998; Magee & Miller, 1997; Crespi, 1995; Goldsmith, 1995; Corbett, 1996; Kiersky, 1996; Isay, 1989), and questioning the dichotomous labels given to heterosexuality, homosexuality, and gender (Goldner, 1991; Schwartz, 1996; D'Ercole, 1996, Butler, 1990). Another representation of recent work focuses on helping gay men and lesbians deal with the traumas experienced due to homophobia in the society at large and in psychotherapy (Drescher, 1999; Blechner, 1995; Frommer, 1994; O'Connor & Ryan, 1993). But the papers in this book focus on the development of a life, the celebration of that life, and the formation of family.

There are notable themes that recur in the papers to follow. One of these themes is that gay and lesbian parenting requires a rethinking of

[Haworth co-indexing entry note]: "Introduction." Glazer, Deborah F. Co-published simultaneously in *Journal of Gay & Lesbian Psychotherapy* (The Haworth Medical Press, an imprint of The Haworth Press, Inc.) Vol. 4, No. 3/4, 2001, pp. 1-6; and: *Gay and Lesbian Parenting* (ed: Deborah F. Glazer, and Jack Drescher) The Haworth Medical Press, an imprint of The Haworth Press, Inc., 2001, pp. 1-6. Single or multiple copies of this article are available from The Haworth Document Delivery Service [1-800-342-9678, 9:00 a.m. - 5:00 p.m. (EST). E-mail address: getinfo@haworthpressinc.com].

our identities. As Sandy Silverman notes, it has been believed that pregnancy (and, one may suppose, the subsequent parenting) has traditionally been viewed as a statement to the world of one's heterosexuality. Conversely, Jack Drescher writes that early identifications in the gay rights movement required relinquishing of parenthood and other emulations of heterosexuality as a way of overcoming the oppression of heterosexual rule. As Drescher puts it, "One had to choose between having children and being gay." As Lee Crespi and Jesse Green note, part of the task of becoming a gay or lesbian parent is overcoming the view of these identifications as being divergent and incompatible. This dilemma of reconciling these identities seems to be a challenge within the individual, within the gay and lesbian communities, and within the society at large. Gay and lesbian parents are navigating their way through family life without the benefit and instruction of the traditional, societally defined archetypal parental roles.

Another theme addressed in many of these papers addresses the question of how to form a family. Green's article begins with the quest for fatherhood, exploring the options of directed sperm donation and adoption. Similarly, Crespi addresses the question of how to acquire the baby as the first question lesbian couples must work through in the development of their families. Unknown donors, known donors, and adoption are all possible avenues, each one having its own intrapsychic and interpersonal meanings and impacts. It becomes clear that biology has not created the question of how to get a baby equally for lesbians and gay men. Carol Buell addresses these questions from a legal standpoint, reviewing the national laws relating to acquiring and securing our families. Both Green and Crespi also raise the question of the meaning of the absent parent–the birth mother or the sperm donor.

At this point, I would like to thank my contributors, and discuss their papers individually. As I mentioned earlier, it is a wonder that this issue came into existence, as it reflects some wonderful changes within psychology, psychoanalysis, and the society at large. (Which should not be confused with the belief that our work is done!) It is also a comment on the fortitude of these authors, many of whom juggle the responsibilities of daily life with parenting responsibilities, full time work, and writing.

In "And Baby Makes Three: A Dynamic Look at Development and Conflict in Lesbian Families," Lee Crespi examines the intrapsychic and interpersonal issues involved as families move from dyadic to triadic. The issue of the triad, the "oedipal" constellation, has been much maligned of late. It has traditionally been viewed as reflective of psychology's rigid adherence to artificially dichotomous gender roles, with winners and losers, and a "successful outcome" is defined as the most narrowly defined representation of procreative heterosexuality. All that aside, any parent of small children with playdate experience will tell you that three is a very hard number. (A difficulty seen in many types of threesomes.) How do couples feel when they decide that two is not enough? What if they don't agree on the need for the third? How do they cope with sharing their partner's attention that used to be all theirs? How do they divide up family roles and functions when they have no similar predecessors upon which to model themselves? Add into the mix all of the old childhood intrapsychic representations of parent/child relationships. It's a wonder any family can make a go of it. But, Crespi finds that a great many lesbian families do succeed. In an important step to understanding our families, Crespi opted not to just evaluate the easily accessible clinical population. Instead, she conducted a study which included anecdotal information obtained through interviews with non-patient families, as well as presenting material from her clinical work. It provides a rounded picture of the difficulties faced by lesbian parents, but also helps us understand the resourceful ways these families survive and thrive.

While Crespi addressed the intrapsychic and interpersonal dynamic issues that affect the growth of the family in the move from a two person unit to a three person unit, I looked at the growth within the individual as a result of the parenting experience. In "Lesbian Motherhood: Restorative Choice or Developmental Imperative?" I explore the ways in which mothering allows for continued intrapsychic development which can result in the reworking of earlier developmental themes. For many women, the experience of mothering can be healing, allowing for the resolution of earlier problems related to the experience of the self, and the capacity to feel loved and genuine. It can also fulfill the adult phase needs for generativity. The concern in the lesbian community, however, is that these increased reproductive options could lead to the belief that becoming a mother is a requirement (i.e., the only option) for continued emotional growth and generativity. A belief that is most assuredly untrue.

Sandy Silverman's "Inevitable Disclosure: Countertransference Dilemmas and the Pregnant Therapist," would seem upon first glance to address a very narrow and specific situation in psychotherapy. In this paper, Silverman discusses her work with patients during her pregnancy. She writes of the assumptions of heterosexuality that some patients, or more correctly, people in general make upon seeing a pregnant woman. For many people, a pregnant lesbian is an oxymoron. Silverman writes of the anxieties of having to address these often confusing self representations with both lesbian and heterosexual patients. But I think this paper transcends the specificity its title implies. Silverman has written a wonderful paper on the inhibitory affects of the therapist's fear of being known by the patient that can result from the therapist's fear of coming out. She notes that it is not always necessary to come out to the patient. In fact, at times that is not what the patient needs. Rather, it is the capacity to be genuine and not afraid to be known that allows for the deepening of the therapeutic work.

Debra Weinstein provides a thoughtful interview with April Martin. Martin has bravely spearheaded the movement to get attention and acceptance for gay and lesbian parents. Martin reflects upon where the movement has been, and where we need to go to assure full equality for the multiplicity of our communities as they move toward the development of family. Later in this volume, Weinstein, a poet and fiction writer, offers powerful poems which allow the reader insight into her own experiences in becoming a mother.

In "Legal Issues Affecting Alternative Families: A Therapist's Primer," Carol Buell provides an excellent overview of the legal issues faced by gay men and lesbians when creating their families. As we see in these articles in this volume, the years of building a family are filled with emotion. Despite the possibility of fear and conflict, it is typically a time of joy and hopefulness. In heterosexual families, the paths toward family formation are more clear, and the legal protections for the family are built into the passages of marriage and parenthood. During this time, gay men and lesbians and the therapists that treat them, need to be aware of the legal options and protections available while forming and maintaining their families.

In "Families of the Lesbian Baby Boom: Maternal Mental Health and Child Adjustment," Charlotte Patterson conducted research that examines the key to well-being in children of lesbians. This study is of vital importance as it counteracts trends seen all too often in family courts, where lesbian parents are allowed to retain custody through the relinquishing of their love relationships, living as single mothers, and curtailing their life style. Patterson found that the mothers in her sample experienced good overall mental health, and that childhood adjustment does not differ based on household constellation. In fact, Patterson found that the best predictor of childhood adjustment was maternal well-being.

I found the next two articles to reflect a fascinating juxtaposition of experiences. Jesse Green's *Velveteen Father* is a memoir of his experiences in becoming a co-father, as well as his lover Andy's quest to fatherhood. The depiction of Andy's attempts to father, which reflect the difficulty many men experience in this quest, is poignant. He writes of the pain and confusion in working through the options available to men, who obviously do not have the same options as lesbians in making their families. He speaks of the suspicion with which many people address men who have the hunger to father, and the guilt inherent in having to take a child from his mother in order to raise him. Green writes of the fear and inadequacy all parents experience, and the ways that differences in temperament and character result in different parenting styles. He expresses the sense of finding a feeling of connectedness through love, family, and religion that can often be lost in the experience of coming out. Green's paper reflects the plight one faces when one feels that without parenting one is not complete, and that parenting can make a gay man feel more real.

Drescher's review offers an insightful historical perspective on the gay male experience, focusing on the time when to be gay and "real" meant the relinquishing of all heterosexual ideals in an attempt to overcome heterosexual oppression. Drescher discusses his own experiences of coming of age at a time men were forced to decide whether they wanted to be gay or have children. A time in which the definitions of "gay" were more clear, and the choices were fewer. But, Drescher speaks of parenting in the same breath as conservatism and religion, equating the excitement these gay men feel about creating family with a return to the right.

The interplay between Green's and Drescher's work reflects what I believe to be an issue in our communities. We have a kind of generation gap. As a result of the intense and successful civil rights work of the prior generations, young gay men and lesbians are afforded greater freedom of choice in their creation of their lives, and this includes the right to parent. Martin says, "It's a radical thing." But, what is radical? Is it choosing to relinquish all the values (some would say constraints) of heterosexuality? Is it saying that we will now live the life that we have been excluded from, including all heterosexual rights, rituals, and responsibilities? Or is it saying that the human experience is varied and vast, and that we have many avenues to growth, generativity, a sense of being loved, and feeling genuine and real. For some, parenting is the way to find it, but for some it is not. And, we finally have the right to choose!

Deborah F. Glazer, PhD

REFERENCES

Blechner, M. (1995). The shaping of psychoanalytic theory and practice by cultural biases about sexuality. In *Disorienting Sexuality: Psychoanalytic Reappraisals of Sexual Identities*, ed. Domenici, T. & Lesser, R.C. New York: Routledge, pp. 265-288.
Bulter, J. (1990). *Gender Trouble: Feminism and the Subversion of Identity:* New York: Routledge.
Corbett, K. (1996). Homosexual boyhood: Notes on girly boys. *Gender and Psychoanalysis*, 1: 429-461.
Crespi, L. (1995). Some thoughts on the role of mourning in the development of a positive lesbian identity. In *Disorienting Sexuality: Psychoanalytic Reappraisals of Sexual Identities*, ed. Domenici, T. & Lesser, R.C. New Yor:, Routledge, pp. 19-32.
D'Ercole, A. (1996). Postmodern ideas about gender and sexuality: The lesbian woman redundancy. *Psychoanalysis and Psychotherapy*, 13:142-152.
Drescher, J. (1999). *Psychoanalytic Therapy and the Gay Man*, New Jersey: The Analytic Press.
Frommer, M.S. (1994). Homosexuality and psychoanalysis: Technical considerations revisited. *Psychoanalytic Dialogues*, 4:215-233.
Goldner, V. (1991). Toward a critical relational theory of gender. *Psychoanalytic Dialogues*, 1:249-272.
Goldsmith, S. (1995). Oedipus or Orestes? Aspects of gender identity in homosexual men. *Psychoanalytic Inquiry*, 15:112-124.
Isay, R. (1989). *Being Homosexual: Gay Men and Their Development*. New York: Farrar, Straus, and Giroux.
Kiersky, S. (1996). Exiled desire: The problem of reality in psychoanalysis and lesbian experience. *Psychoanalysis and Psychotherapy*, 13:130-141.
Magee, M. & Miller, D.C. (1997). *Lesbian Lives: Psychoanalytic Narratives Old and New*. New Jersey: The Analytic Press.
O'Connor, N. & Ryan, J. (1993) *Wild Desires and Mistaken Identities: Lesbianism and Psychoanalysis*, New York: Columbia University Press.
Schwartz, A.E. (1998). *Sexual Subjects: Lesbians, Gender, and Psychoanalysis*. New York: Routledge.
Schwartz, D. (1996). Questioning the social construction of gender and sexual orientation. *Gender and Psychoanalysis*, 1:249-260.

And Baby Makes Three:
A Dynamic Look at Development
and Conflict in Lesbian Families

Lee Crespi, CSW

SUMMARY. When a couple decides to have a child its members experience a resurgence of earlier intrapsychic issues. For lesbian couples the lack of a social construct to guide them in family formation brings an added challenge. Through personal interviews and clinical examples this paper explores some of the ways in which these intrapsychic issues may manifest, both as conflict and as potential for growth. *[Article copies available for a fee from The Haworth Document Delivery Service: 1-800-342-9678. E-mail address: <getinfo@haworthpressinc.com> Website: <http://www.Haworth Press.com> © 2001 by The Haworth Press, Inc. All rights reserved.]*

KEYWORDS. Lesbians, families, motherhood, triangulation, donor insemination, adoption

All happy families are alike; each unhappy family is unhappy in its own way.

–Leo Tolstoy, *Anna Karenina*

When two become three with the arrival of a child, each parent's Oedipal drama is revisited, with its attendant conflicts and potential

---

Lee Crespi is on the Executive Board, Psychoanalytic Psychotherapy Study Center, and Supervisor, Institute for Contemporary Psychotherapy, both in New York City. The author is also in private practice.

Address correspondence to: Lee Crespi, CSW, 153 Waverly Place, 10th Floor, New York, NY 10014 (E-mail: LCrespi@worldnet.att.net).

[Haworth co-indexing entry note]: "And Baby Makes Three: A Dynamic Look at Development and Conflict in Lesbian Families." Crespi, Lee. Co-published simultaneously in *Journal of Gay & Lesbian Psychotherapy* (The Haworth Medical Press, an imprint of The Haworth Press, Inc.) Vol. 4, No. 3/4, 2001, pp. 7-29; and: *Gay and Lesbian Parenting* (ed: Deborah F. Glazer, and Jack Drescher) The Haworth Medical Press, an imprint of The Haworth Press, Inc., 2001, pp. 7-29. Single or multiple copies of this article are available from The Haworth Document Delivery Service [1-800-342-9678, 9:00 a.m. - 5:00 p.m. (EST). E-mail address: getinfo@haworthpressinc.com].

resolutions. Long before their child is faced with issues of triangulation, the parents are confronted with their own feelings of jealousy, competition and exclusion. While some on the psychoanalytic right may argue that this paradigm cannot be applied to a lesbian family,[1] which, by its very nature, defies the Oedipal situation, I disagree. On an intrapsychic level, regardless of the couple's sexual orientation, internal objects continue to play out various themes in relation to the desire to possess one or the other parent, apart from the genders of the actual individuals (Butler, 1995). And while some on the post-modern left may discount the validity of the Oedipal construct altogether, I would likewise disagree, and argue that such a paradigm is still a functional and potent tool to explain and organize some very real and inevitable dynamics of parent/child relationships.

The availability of donor sperm and the increased acceptance of lesbians by adoption agencies and courts has changed the complexion of life for lesbians of this generation (Glazer, 1998; Crespi, 1997). It is now close to two decades since lesbians began, *as lesbians*, to become mothers. We have gone from a generation for whom parenting was only an option if they had been previously married, to one for whom childrearing has become not only an option but, in some cases, an imperative.

As a psychotherapist working extensively with lesbians and as a lesbian mother myself, I have become increasingly aware of the need to articulate some of the dynamic issues, Oedipal and otherwise, faced by new lesbian families. In discussions with colleagues and other parents, within and without the lesbian community, I have become aware of certain recurrent concerns. "How do two women decide how they will create a family, and what is the impact of this decision? What role, if any, does biology play in the relationships between family members? How can we understand problems of jealousy and exclusion? How do roles evolve when both parents are women? Can a child really have two mommies?" (My son's friends often ask this last question, as well.) And, perhaps, most important from a clinical standpoint, what determines why some couples have difficulty, or even fail, in creating viable family units?

I hope in this paper to offer some formulations based on a number of sources: individual psychoanalysis and couples therapy with my own patients as well as cases shared with me by colleagues and supervisees. In addition, in order to expand the representation from an exclusively clinical sample, I have conducted interviews with other lesbian mothers in my personal and professional acquaintance, and conferred with the director of Centerkids.[2] By posting a notice on the Internet I was also able to speak to and interview another 15 families from across the United States about their experiences as lesbians raising children together. My sample was small, and it was socio-economically homogeneous, predominantly white,[3] middle-class, professionals. However, by including a non-clinical as well as a clinical population, my hope is that it more accurately reflects a balance than would a purely clinical sampling. This was by no means intended to be quantitative research, but rather an attempt to draft a beginning map of the different ways that lesbian families develop structurally, functionally and psychodynamically. In so doing, I hope to identify some of the developmental problems that face these families, in order to provide a beginning guide to helping families in conflict.

The experience of becoming a mother is, by its very nature, regressive. (Winnicott, 1956). The mother-to-be experiences a loosening of her defenses (Blos, 1985), which brings about a repetition of intrapsychic processes originating in her own infancy. This regression provides an opportunity for her to revisit and resolve not only Oedipal but also primary oral conflicts with her own mother (Benedek, 1959). In this way, the mothering experience is growth enhancing and reparative (Frankfeldt, 1999; Glazer, 1998). At the same time, this regression may lower the woman's capacity to negotiate the needs of her partner when they conflict with her own. Heterosexual couples encounter the same regressive pulls, but the conflicts manifest differently because of the socially structured gender roles. Also, because of the lack of social support and of available identificatory objects, lesbian couples lack a roadmap for understanding and resolving conflicts which arise as a result of these regressive forces.

At this stage, the opportunity presented to rework earlier issues can be profound and very positive. One woman reported that when her son was born, she was surprised to find that, although she had always wanted a daughter, she felt secretly proud, almost smug, to have a son. The power deriving from the archaic social status of being mother to a son, as well as the opportunity for cross-gender identification, made her feel very powerful and complete. At the same time, her feelings toward her partner deepened considerably, and although her partner had obviously not impregnated her, she felt as if symbolically she had done so, by making it possible for her to have this experience. Another woman described how she felt that her internalized homophobia was ameliorated by a sense that "if God is willing to allow me to have this child, then it must be really all right for me to be a lesbian."

There are specific points in the process of having children at which the greatest potential for both conflict and growth may arise. These are (1) the decision to have a child at all (2) deciding *who* should bear or adopt the child, and (3) the establishment of parental roles.

STAGE ONE: LET'S HAVE A BABY!

The first challenge on the path to parenthood for lesbian couples is in coming to the decision to have children at all. For most of the lesbians in this study, this was a decision they had considered for many years before settling on a course of action. They felt like pioneers, and had to readjust their thinking about themselves in order to fit a new prototype.

Internalized homophobia was an obstacle faced by some in contemplating whether to have children. As one woman described it, she felt that, as a lesbian, she was not entitled to a child.

> I had assumed that as a lesbian, children were out of the picture for me. When my partner began raising the issue, I resisted at first. But then I began to examine my life and I felt, well, I've achieved my career, we have a house, a nice life, now what? I realized that I not only had room in my life for children but I began to reconsider getting older and *not* doing it. With a child, I would be able to pass on all the things and experiences I have had, and I hopefully could help bring a new person in the world who liked to laugh, experience things, meet people, and would be a contributing member to society.

While many of the couples that I interviewed had arrived at their decision jointly, just as many had been divided at first. For most of those couples who proceeded and now had children, the difference between the partners had not been experienced so much as a source of conflict, but rather, as tension over coming to terms with differences, or pressure to resolve unconscious issues related to becoming a parent. They described a sense of process and of one member of the couple persuading the other over time. Of the partners who initially did not want children, most related changing their minds initially out of a feeling of love for their partners, empathy for the strength of her wish for a child, and then a shift in their internal awareness of a need for something generative in their own lives.[4]

In my clinical practice, I have worked with many lesbian couples who are in the stage of struggling with the decision to have a child. In many cases, like the ones above, there is a strong feeling of empathy between the partners, and a concern that one partner will be unhappy if the other prevails. In other cases, the early issues that are triggered by the prospect of motherhood may cause the couple to polarize and may ignite conflicts centered around Oedipal or pre-Oedipal concerns. For example, the woman who wants a child may experience her partner's opposition as that of a withholding parent, or of a jealous mother who wishes to deny her daughter's fertility. She may resort to threats and exhortation, with little or no regard for the subjective experience of her partner. Her investment in having a child may be so great that she is unable to hear serious objections that her partner raises. She may be unable to face the possibility of loss which may result if she must choose between her partner and her wish to have a child. At the same time, a woman who feels she is being unduly pressured to agree to parenthood may re-experience fears of abandonment or of being re-placed by a younger sibling. She may feel competitive with her part-ner's wish for a child, and resent not being "enough." Conflicts in her identification with her own parents may contribute to reluctance to assume a parental role for fear of failing at one. A strong need for an exclusively dyadic[5] relationship may be threatened by the partner's wish for a child. This may be the result of an overly symbiotic tie to her own mother, which was never sufficiently resolved, or conversely, insufficient nurture from her mother that may have left her in a state of object hunger.[6]

Example

Jessica and Holly sought therapy to resolve their conflict about having a child. Jessica very much wanted to bear a child of her own. Holly feared that if Jessica bore a child she would feel emotionally abandoned by her. Her own childhood had been characterized by a serious lack of adequate nurturing and she felt unready to be a parent. In reaction to feeling pressured by Jessica she suggested that as a compromise they could adopt a child, thereby eliminating the biological bond between Jessica and the baby and providing an opportunity for Holly to feel less excluded. Jessica did not feel that this was an adequate solution, as she wanted very much to bear a child herself, both for the experience of pregnancy and for the genetic connection. She alternated between being understanding of Holly's fear and feeling angry with her for her inability to support her. As the therapist attempted to explore their respective feelings regarding having a child, the couple continued to try coming up with concrete plans to bypass the painful emotional impasse in which they found themselves. At one point, they considered having Holly donate the egg and Jessica carry the baby. Jessica then vetoed this as too complicated. This caused Holly to feel that Jessica was trying to maintain her primary connection to the baby, which reinforced her fears of abandonment and exclusion. At another point, they agreed to adopt, but then Jessica again retreated, saying it was too costly. These repeated attempts to come up with a solution that bypassed their feelings served as a defense against experiencing those feelings. Holly was torn between her fear of losing Jessica's love to a baby, or losing her altogether. Defending against powerful feelings of loss, Jessica was reluctant to give up her desire for a biological child of her own thus reinforcing Holly's feeling that Jessica was not going to be able to include her emotionally after the baby was born. Both women had issues related to unresolved mourning which made it difficult for them to stay with the feelings of loss that each faced as they worked through this decision.

Example

Amy and Therese had been together three years when they sought therapy to resolve their impasse about having a baby. Already in her late thirties, Amy had been clear from the outset of their relationship that she wanted a child. Therese had agreed enthusiastically at that time but later recanted claiming that the intoxication of romance had clouded her judgement. Amy alternated between being furious at feeling duped and believing that she could cajole Therese to reconsider. She could see that Therese loved children and enjoyed being around them. Because of her ambivalence, Therese would allow herself to be persuaded and then back off angrily. In couple sessions, Therese was able to explain clearly and effectively her genuine concerns about parenting. A number of issues emerged. Therese had a strong negative identification with her father who had been irresponsible but charismatic. She saw herself, like him, as a "free spirit" and longed to travel around the world. She feared that a baby would tie her down, as five children had tied down her mother. At the same time, she was afraid she would be a failure as a parent as she felt her father to be. She had grown up in poverty and felt she needed to provide a "perfect" home for her child. As a lesbian, she felt she would be unable to do that because she would be burdening a child by bringing it into a world that didn't accept its parents' homosexuality.

Amy, the oldest child in her large family, had always wanted children and had always involved herself with women who needed nurturing and caretaking. She had believed that Therese was different and was able to be an equal partner. That had been true until recently, but now she wondered if Therese was regressing to being a child in their relationship. In addition, Amy tended to minimize conflict in an effort to defend against her anger. As she realized that Therese's objections were genuine she became increasingly depressed. Amy's depression, recapitulating as it did Therese's mother's unhappiness, made Therese more anxious and doubtful about their ability to raise a child. The very qualities that had attracted her to Amy, her stability and responsibility, now felt controlling and stifling. As Therese was able to express her misgivings about parenthood without Amy repeatedly countering every thought with an argument or reassurance, she began to move through her fears and to recognize their genetic origins. She began to soften in her resistance and to acknowledge that she was afraid of feeling deprived again, as she had as a child. Amy began to better hear what Therese was saying and to see that she couldn't get what she wanted by pushing. At the same time, she recognized that her depression was the result of her own refusal to face the possibility that she would have to choose between having a baby or being with Therese. As Amy stopped pushing, Therese not only stopped resisting but became actively supportive and the two have now begun exploring their options for having a baby.

These examples reflect some of the ways that earlier issues may get reactivated in the process of negotiating the decision as to whether to become parents. In the first case, the inability to face the painful feelings that were surfacing led the couple to repeatedly try to fix the problem without solving it. In the second case, the couple's ability to examine all of their feelings openly led to their successfully resolving their conflict with neither partner feeling coerced.

STAGE TWO: HOW TO DO IT

The next point at which issues of conflict and competition may arise for prospective lesbian parents is in deciding by what method they will bring a child into their lives. For some, the lack of societal legitimacy of the lesbian relationship itself heightens the importance that the children serve to legitimize the marriage. For this reason, many lesbian couples opt to take turns conceiving a child using the same donor so that the family will be balanced and everyone related to each other through this biological connection. For adoptive parents, the legal sanction of the courts in allowing both parents to adopt (in those states where second parent adoption is open to lesbians) is the closest thing to a marriage license that lesbians can achieve.

Donor Insemination (DI)

The choice to bear a child through donor insemination was the favored alternative of most lesbians with whom I have spoken, reflective of a prevailing desire to be biologically related to the child. When both partners feel strongly about having a genetic connection to the child, and wish to mitigate a perceived potential for imbalance in the family, efforts may be made to create genetic ties to both women. This may be done through the use of sperm donated by a relative of one woman to impregnate the other or through egg donation by one partner to the other. More frequently, couples plan to each bear a child consecutively, preferably using the same sperm donor. Another reason expressed for choosing donor insemination (DI) is a desire to have the physical experience of pregnancy and childbirth. Again, if this is an experience that both women desire, the decision is made, when possible, to each bear a child. Negative feelings about adoption, such as concern over the danger of having an adopted child taken away, and to a lesser degree, social prejudices about adoption are a factor for some women, as well as is the comparative ease of getting pregnant[7] vs. adopting a child. Since, both women have the possibility of becoming pregnant, infertility in one partner does not rule out the likelihood of a birth.

At this stage, if both partners are believed to be fertile, the question of *who* will bear the child is the one that distinguishes lesbian couples from heterosexuals, and that may introduce a competitive dimension. For many couples, the decision is made pragmatically based on either inclination or age with no conflict or hesitation. However, when *both* women have an intense desire to mother, rivalry may occur over who conceives (Glazer 1998). Issues of competition may then arise, that if not addressed may be carried into the family well after the child arrives laying the groundwork for later difficulties. If one woman is unable to conceive, the competitive issues may be compounded even further.

Example

Claire had always wanted to have a child but her partner Lori had been initially somewhat reluctant. She felt preoccupied by her unmet professional goals, and felt unprepared to assume the responsibilities of a family. This was an ongoing area of conflict for the couple for a number of years. Then, following the death of her mother, Lori began longing for a child of her own. Since she was also older than Claire, they agreed that she would conceive first, and that Claire would then follow a few years later. Although Claire agreed to this arrangement, she felt that she had been preempted. When Lori was slow to conceive, she felt impatient, as though she were "waiting in the wings." Once their first child was born, these feelings receded to the background. It wasn't until after their second child was born, birthed by Claire herself, that they reemerged into consciousness.

Infertility

Infertility in any woman who wants a child brings with it feelings of loss and inadequacy. For lesbians, it raises added issues that are somewhat different than for heterosexual women. When one partner clearly wants to have the experience of childbearing and the primacy that comes with being a biological mother but tries unsuccessfully to conceive, the fact that her partner does conceive can be a mixed blessing. The infertile partner needs to mourn the loss of her childbearing potential, but her partner, or she herself, may be eager to get on with trying to have a child. This would be similar to the experience of a heterosexual woman with one important divergence. The heterosexual woman may have other options for becoming a mother but she does not have a spouse waiting in the wings to do the very thing that she has been unable to do.

At times, some lesbians may be found to have an inadequate and marred internal representation of a gendered self (Schwartz, 1998). There are a number of intrapsychic factors that may contribute to this including ambivalence toward and disidentification with her own mother, a history of feeling defective as a result of early awareness of being different, conflicting familial attitudes toward women and internalization of negative cultural perceptions about lesbians. Failure to conceive can compound these feelings of failure as a woman and make the mourning process more problematic.

Example

Denise and Abby had been together for several years when they decided jointly that they wanted a child. Abby had a strong desire to bear a child. Denise, who loved children and looked forward to being a parent, felt less of a need to experience pregnancy and childbirth, or even to be biologically connected to the child. However, when it became evident that Abby was having difficulty conceiving, a variety of problems surfaced in the couple. Denise had always been the accommodating member of the couple who internalized her anger and dissatisfactions while Abby was far more vocal and assertive of her needs. Denise's mother had been very demanding and suffered numerous somatic problems during Denise's childhood. Denise had catered to her mother and maintained a close relationship with her by repressing her own needs and anger. Denise found herself again playing the supporting role to Abby's emotional distress. This was then compounded when Abby began taking fertility drugs that contributed to her becoming even more emotionally demanding. Denise began to grow increasingly resentful. She offered to try to get pregnant but Abby was not ready to give up her attempts. Denise felt wounded by Abby's refusal to let her try to conceive. She began to experience Abby as the Oedipal mother who would not let her assert her own strivings, and as the narcissistic mother who had to be centerstage at any cost. She felt that if Abby loved her she would accept Denise's baby as an adequate alternative to having one of her own. Abby, in turn, felt conflicted. She recognized the logic in Denise's offer but was really not ready to give up trying to conceive. She came from a very competitive family and was one of three sisters, both of whom already had children. As a lesbian, she felt that no matter how much success she achieved in her life she was always at a disadvantage. Having a baby would be an achievement that was important to her in her relationship with her family.

Abby's desire to bear a child herself was too pressing for her to relinquish. Her strong need to be the bearer of the child and therefore in her mind the primary parent made her resent Denise's failure to continue to acquiesce. As a result she was unable to fully articulate to Denise just what it meant to her to fail at this endeavor. In some ways, Denise was correct in her perception that Abby was focused on her own narcissistic and competitive needs and not on the relationship. The tension in the couple continued to mount and they grew more distant. After two years Abby became pregnant, but the couple broke up before the baby was born.

Example

A second couple, Jo and Kathleen, also struggled with infertility. Jo, who had the stronger desire to bear a child ultimately passed the torch to Kathleen. Jo was able to go through the experience of intense mourning, which took her several years, while at the same time embracing the idea of Kathleen having their child, despite the pain it evoked. Her desire to have a child in their family was stronger than her ambivalence about Kathleen being the one to bear it. Because of greater access to her own grief, and the opportunity to work it through in her own analysis, she was able to separate the issues. Her wish for a child propelled her forward. Once their son was born, she ultimately became the primary parent, as Kathleen resumed her more demanding work schedule while Jo was able to cut hers back. She recalls that in the beginning she felt a great need to let people know that Jake was both of theirs, but adds, "time heals many wounds." Now ten years old, and with a younger sibling, Jake has moved back and forth between the two of them for differing needs at different stages. Jo is very clear that with both of their boys, she was the mother of the early years, while Kathleen is the parent who engages in older child activities, and being less at home, is experienced as the more exciting one.

Donor Selection

The question of whether to use a known or unknown donor often introduces issues related to triangulation. Among couples who have rejected the idea of having a known donor, most have stated very clearly their concern about having a third adult, and a man in particular, disrupt the equilibrium and primacy of their family constellation. A frequent worry was of jealousy and the fear that the non-biological mother would have less status than would the donor. Some couples, out of a desire for the child to have a male figure in their lives, choose to use known donors. For these couples, the experience has ranged from wanting the donor to be more involved, to, less often, finding themselves in legal conflict over the rights of the various parties. In most cases, in families who do engage known donors, the choice has been a successful one. Families have even been extended to include the partner of the donor as well, such that the child has two mommies *and* two daddies.

In regard to issues of triangulation the sperm donor is a very important figure whose presence is always felt even if he is unknown.

> The donor presents many faces to the lesbian couple. He is at once their liberator, because he offers them the freedom to have children . . . He, in the ultimate anonymous form, offers them total control over the destiny of their child . . . If known, [he] can either be a cooperative, interested important adjunct to the child or he can be perceived as an intrusive controlling interfering person. At the worst, the donor could be a legal threat to the vulnerable lesbian couple. (Baran & Pannor, 1989)

In addition, the donor carries half the child's genetic history. His appearance, character traits, temperament may all be evident in the child, making his presence felt in the family despite his absence. As a man, he may represent a threat to the non-biological mother as having the ability to do what she cannot, i.e., impregnate her partner and be the child's father. He may be loved as the giver of a gift of life, and/or resented as the necessary but unwanted member of the family.

Adoption

Lesbians that had chosen adoption did so for a variety of reasons. For many, DI had been their first choice, but neither partner had been able to conceive. Of these women, some experienced very strong reactions of loss, as I have described in the previous section. Others, though, seemed to feel that having a child was their main concern. They did not choose to enter into fertility treatments or other extra measures but moved readily to the adoption process.

Some lesbians chose adoption as their first choice. The reasons for this included one or more of the following:

1. The wish for both women to have an equal connection to the child, in order to mitigate feelings of competition and exclusiv-

ity, which they felt would not be possible if only one of them was biologically related to it.

2. Socio/political reasons, i.e., a sense that adoption offered them a chance to contribute something by providing a home to a child who needed one.
3. Personal experience with adoption, as for example, being adopted themselves.
4. Family history of genetic problems such hemophilia.
5. The ability, when adopting through an agency, to choose the gender of the child.

There are some important choices to be made in the adoption process, but the choices that bear directly on the couple's relationship include deciding who will be the adoptive parent, since there are few places where a lesbian couple can adopt together, and decisions about race or ethnicity that may be relevant to the couple's demographics. For example, a number of couples with whom I spoke were of mixed race or ethnicity, and made a point of seeking a child who would reflect either both of their backgrounds or the background of the mother of minority status. The issue of who would be the legal parent appeared to be far less loaded as a competitive issue than in pregnancy/birth situations. This may be because of the existence of the adopted child's birth mother who represents the ultimate rival for the child's love and loyalty in the mind of the adoptive parents. Just as the sperm donor is the additional family member who may be loved and resented simultaneously, so, in adoption, the birth mother (and, to a lesser degree the birth father), may be loved as the giver of life, but resented as a potential competitor.

Overall, the process of sorting through the various options for creating a family, when done reflectively, can be very growth enhancing. Each woman must examine her fantasies and expectations of what she wants from a child and from having a family. In addition to competitive issues, various other dynamics may come into play as well. Internalized homophobia, for example, may come up unexpectedly. One woman explained to me that she felt that as a lesbian she did not have the right to bring a child into the world, but that if she adopted, it was all right, because the child was already in the world. Yet, another woman said that she felt she had to give birth herself rather than adopt because "who would be willing to give their baby to a lesbian couple?"

STAGE THREE: WHO'S GETTING UP? ESTABLISHING ROLES

Once these fundamental decisions have been made and a child enters their lives, the next challenge for the lesbian couple may arise in the process of finding and developing their respective roles as parents. Much of the preparatory work is done during the pregnancy or the wait for the adoptive child. During this time, the couple begins, through fantasy as well as in concrete ways to share their expectations and identify their needs in relation to the new family constellation. Preparing the child's room, selecting a name, announcing the impending arrival to family and coworkers, or simply lying in bed whispering together in anticipation and awe as expectant parents have done since the beginning of time. All provide opportunities to begin the work of reconfiguring the new family and finding each member's internally resonant role. For most couples this process unfolds smoothly, as each woman finds herself gravitating toward the role that suits her disposition and resonates with her own parental identifications. When these roles are complementary, each partner accommodates the other in a fluid and mutually supportive way.

Complementary roles need not imply that lesbian families divide up the parenting roles according to the traditional heterosexual model. In fact, while some couples do employ this model, e.g., one parent staying at home and assuming the bulk of the domestic responsibilities and the other working and providing financial support, most do not. In most lesbian families, both parents work either full or part-time. They allocate activities such as getting ready in the morning, putting the child to bed, getting up during the night, feeding, and playing, more on the basis of either personal proclivities, such as who can fall back to sleep more easily when being awakened from a sound sleep, or they merely trade off. One couple reports that their son is so used to them alternating getting up with him in the morning that he pops his head into their bedroom and calls out gaily "Who's getting up?"

Of greater concern to many lesbians, particularly when considering DI is whether the biological mother[8] will, a priori, have the stronger bond with the child, but that has not been found to be the case. In fact, many of the couples interviewed, found that the co-mother when actively and fully engaged in caregiving had the potential for an equal or even stronger bond. In some cases, the biological mother returned to work to a more demanding schedule, leaving the partner the opportunity to spend more time with the child as with Jo in the example above. In other cases, the partner's personality style propelled her to take a more active role, either because she was less anxious or temperamentally more attracted to caring for an infant. When breastfeeding could be alternated with bottle feeding the partner was able to share, albeit differently, in the early feeding experience. One couple described how one partner would get up in the middle of the night and bring the baby to the other's breast, thus allowing the nursing mother to remain partially asleep, and allowing the partner to participate in a shared experience. In general, where deeper conflicts were not evident, when the non-birth mother chose, and was permitted, to take an equal role in most daily routines, the child appeared to bond relatively equally to both. When preferences *were* shown, they alternated and shifted over time, as would be expected given the normal stages of child development. In these families, when competitive feelings did arise, they were usually transient and were mitigated by a capacity for emotional identification by each woman with her partner's experience, as well as by the inevitable shifting of preferences within the child.

When one partner assumed the primary nurturing role, whether the biological or the co-parent, the child showed a clear preference for that parent. This was also the case in adoptive families where one woman was the legal parent and one was not. In studies of infants of primary nurturing fathers, even among those that had been breast-fed, the babies all demonstrated a decided preference and stronger bond to the father, to the extent of developing similar personality traits and interests (Pruet, 1983). Research substantiates that "the child's response to either parent . . . is more a function of the nature of the parent-child interaction than of a biological predisposition" (Kotelchuck, 1976). When the primary nurturing parent is also the biological mother, there is more of a potential for feelings of exclusion to arise and for the non-biological mother to feel peripheral.

It is not uncommon for some infants to demonstrate not simply a preference for one parent, but rejecting behavior toward the other parent at various stages of development. Along with possible constitutional factors, Abelin (1980) postulates that there is an early recognition of the triangular family structure long before the Oedipal phase that the infant responds to in a variety of ways, including by trying to separate the parents. We would also expect that the unconscious needs of the parents are acted out by the infant's relationship to each of them and at the very least reinforced by the parents' needs. If one parent needs to maintain a symbiotic closeness with the child, the other parent, rather than being able to facilitate the child's separation, may be experienced as a threat. If the child is then unable to experience ambivalent feelings toward the primary parent because they are a threat to that parent, he may split them off to the other parent resulting in a relationship characterized by anger and rejection. When the choice of who will bear the child is reflective of an already existing unconscious conflict in the couple's needs in regard to the child, it may well be played out in the roles that develop after the child is born.

The non-biological, non-caregiving, lesbian mother is at a triple disadvantage. She has neither given birth to, nor is she the primary nurturer of the child. In addition, as a lesbian she must establish her role in relationship to the child and to the mother/child dyad without any socially defined constructs that could legitimize her status in the family. She may, in fact, have no legal standing in relation to the child. She has no role models with whom to identify, and receives little direction or reinforcement from the social milieu, which often does not recognize her as a parent at all (Tasker, 1997). Much depends on the individual woman's ability to address the conflicts and anxieties that are stimulated by this scenario.

Competition and Exclusion

While most couples move smoothly into the phase of establishing parental roles, for others this can also be a time of unexpected dissonance. Glazer (1998) has discussed the phenomenon of "Competitive Mothering" as follows:

> For lesbians who are co-parenting, who may have unresolved oedipal issues, and who may not feel adequately female, issues regarding competition can be a likely source of distress. . . . In birth and adoption situations, one woman may be identified as the 'true mother.' The non-biological/non-legal mother may face unexpected feelings of anger and rejection related to breast feeding, signing for medical treatment, etc. (p. 147)

A strong desire to mother may oftentimes be accompanied by an equally strong sense of entitlement to be the primary parent (Crawford, 1987). This may derive from a woman's identification with her own mother, and an internal psychological representation of *Mother* that does not resonate with being in a secondary position in relation to the child. In addition, women are socialized to expect to be the primary nurturers, and there are no social constructs for women, as there are for men, to organize their feelings of exclusion or rejection when the child shows a strong preference for one parent over the other Traditionally, the role of the father in the early years of a child's life, has been seen as supporting and protecting the mother/child dyad (Winnicott, 1956), fostering exploration and disentangling the child from the symbiotic tie to the mother (Mahler, 1966), and facilitating gender identification. Research into families where the father is the primary caretaker (Pruet, 1983) demonstrates that these fathers can nurture and bond as deeply as mothers and suggests that this is because these fathers have strong positive identifications with their own nurturing mothers. Likewise, if a lesbian is able to call upon a positive identification with her own father, she may be able to assume a role of supporter, stimulator, and mediator without conflict.

For a lesbian who has disidentified with her mother (Schwartz, 1998) but is conflicted about identifying with her father, this ambiguous role has the potential to stir up feelings of inadequacy. She may feel that she is failing as a woman if she is not the primary nurturer. This will be compounded if she has also been unable to conceive. She may feel her gender identity threatened by being perceived as being in the traditional "dad" role. If her relationship to her father is conflicted, she could lack access to a positive internal model with whom to identify. Since there are so few, if any, archetypes in our culture to support either a woman in the role of co-parent (or a man as primary nurturer), she will have few places to turn for validation and confirmation.

Example

Carla is the non-biological mother of Jake. She has a soft-spoken and somewhat tentative style, despite her underlying depth and tenacity. Susan is Jake's biological mother. She is outgoing and bold, with a warm and generous nature. When Jake was first born, Carla helped at the delivery, and having had a great deal of experience handling babies, was the more active during early infancy. Susan had difficulty with her milk so Jake was bottle fed making Carla's access to him even greater. This quickly changed as Carla resumed working and

Susan spent more time at home with Jake. As Jake's bond with Susan, his biological mother, intensified, Carla felt increasingly on the periphery. "I hung back. I guess it's my nature. I didn't feel entitled, so I deferred." Lacking a sense of entitlement to Jake's affection, and feeling ambiguity about her new role as a lesbian co-parent, Carla reacted in an ego-syntonic deferential manner. Susan continued to actively encourage Carla's participation and Carla clearly bonded with Jake, having a definite role in his life as the more calm and separate parent. She felt very close to him but always felt that he was Susan's baby. Three years later, when she gave birth to Lily, she began to realize that it was hers and Susan's personalities that determined the children's relationship to each of them. Although Carla breast fed Lily, and was the one to get up with her during the night, Susan continued to be the primary caretaker to both children, even after she herself returned to working fulltime. "Susan is warmer and stronger than I am, she gets right in there and doesn't hold back. If Lily showed a preference for me, it didn't bother her, she just made a space for herself. That's how she is." As a result, Carla no longer has the feeling that their children belong to one or the other of them. In retrospect she recognizes that she accepted a secondary role out of her own anxiety, a degree of internalized homophobia, and because she had no models of how a lesbian family could be configured.

Example

From the outset of their relationship, Ingrid and Joanne were very much in agreement about wanting children. They went through the stages of deciding about method and choosing a donor without conflict. They each planned on having a child utilizing the same sperm donor. They agreed that Ingrid would conceive first, as she was older, more eager and less anxious about it. Both women worked full time and employed in-home childcare, although Ingrid's job permitted her to have more time at home. Early on, their son, William showed a strong preference for Ingrid, his biological mother, "so much so," says Ingrid, "that it was embarrassing. When you have two moms, you both expect to be primary. What do you do?" Despite Ingrid's efforts to bring the two together, Joanne began to feel a sense of failure, as William increasingly rejected her. At one point, they consulted a child specialist who assured them that his behavior was normal and that this occurred frequently in heterosexual families as well.

This did not seem to assuage Joanne's sense of hurt and rejection. At the same time, Ingrid felt guilty, "the preferred mother gets a lot of power." She did not feel good about the triangulation but felt powerless to change it. She encouraged Joanne to get pregnant herself. When she did become pregnant, she was surprised to see that William reacted very strongly. He became fearful that she was going to abandon him. It may have seemed to him that he had destroyed their relationship through his anger, and that she was going to replace him with another child. It became much clearer to both Ingrid and Joanne that William's attachment to Joanne was far greater than they had realized, but it was an attachment that was expressed through rejection and negativity.

These examples illustrate the power that the child's natural preferences may have in triggering anxiety and competitiveness in the parental couple. In each situation, the parents' confusion about their own roles contributed to the confusion caused by the natural temperament of the child and/or the parents. In both cases, however, the biological mother's commitment to supporting her partner and including her greatly ameliorated the situation.

DYADIC vs. TRIADIC

More problematic than competition between the two mothers, is what I have come to understand as a dyadic vs. triadic problem. This appears when one (or both[9]) of the women has a strong unresolved need for a two-person relationship that supercedes her ability to enter into a three-person relationship. This may be the result of an overly symbiotic tie to her own mother, which was never sufficiently resolved, or conversely, insufficient nurture from her mother that has left her in a state of object hunger. The introduction of a child to the couple restimulates these dyadic needs and destabilizes the bond, resulting in the exclusion of one partner. This may manifest itself in a variety of ways. For example, either partner may become overly critical of the other's parenting, and try to control all situations involving the child. One woman accounted that in retrospect she believes that as the birth-mother she devalued her partner's role, and tried to render her impotent because she felt such a strong need to experience the kind of early intense bond that she had missed in her own childhood. At the same time, her partner longed for the same dyadic bond, and felt deep resentment at being excluded. This was further compounded by having tried and been unable to conceive a child herself, which made her feel like failure, and led to feelings of destructive envy toward her partner's ability to bear a child. As discussed earlier, the regressive experience that accompanies motherhood can be quite disorganizing and may lead to reemergence of powerful early needs that interfere with each woman's ability to tolerate her partner's needs in relation to her and the child. Instead, she may see them as a threat and her partner as an interloper who is trying to come between her and the child.[10]

Example

Lorraine and Trish discussed the possibility of having a child for many years. Lorraine's reluctance was based primarily on her anxiety that she and Trish would lose their close connection, which she felt it had been her role to protect. After several years of discussion and a great deal of thought, Lorraine began to find the prospect of raising a child increasingly appealing. By the time they decided to go ahead with it, Lorraine was very excited and determined to share equally in the parenting. However, almost immediately after the birth of their son, Taylor, problems began to arise. While Trish remained at home with the baby, Lorraine returned to her busy career. Although they had planned to share the feeding of Taylor, he rejected the bottle, making it impossible for Lorraine to feed him. Lorraine began to feel increasing excluded from the dyad. At the same time, the critical illness of one of her siblings began to press on her time and energy drawing her further away from her partner and their baby. For Trish the experience of giving birth and nursing a baby was a profoundly reparative one, particularly in relation to lifelong feelings of alienation from her own body. In addition, the regression activated by caring for an infant reawakened her symbiotic ties to her own mother. She needed Lorraine's support and resented her unavailability, while at the same time, she unconsciously found ways to keep her from getting close to their son. For example, despite Lorraine's objections she continued to breast feed him far longer than they had originally planned. Taylor's bond to Trish intensified, while his relationship to Lorraine became more rejecting.

Lorraine, in turn, found her own difficulties with triangles and with being on the outside to become increasingly troubling. Her reaction to the seemingly exclusive bond between Trish and Taylor was to capitulate angrily and retreat even further. The family became rigidly polarized, with Lorraine on the outside alternately trying to break in and then withdrawing in defeat. Trish was left feeling pulled at and attacked by Lorraine, and felt that she had to protect Taylor from Lorraine's criticism and efforts to come between them. This dynamic continued for several years with little improvement and eventually led to the couple's separation.

CONCLUSION

Becoming a parent is a major developmental challenge. The decline in extended family supports, the increase in two working parent families, the high rate of divorce, and the overall lack of social and political valuation of parenting greatly adds to the burden faced by all prospective parents in our society. For lesbian families, there are additional social and political obstacles that must be overcome, including lack of recognition, absence of legal sanctions, prejudice, and lack of role models, to name a few (Crawford, 1987). At each major crossroad in the process of family formation–including the decision *whether* to become parents, *how* to become parents and *what* shape the parental roles will take–there is a convergence of developmental and sociopolitical issues with relational and intrapsychic dynamics which will determine whether the couple can successfully negotiate these issues or whether they will be stymied by conflict.

Research has shown that lesbian and gay parents, because of these added hurdles, tend to do an extensive amount of soul searching before undertaking parenthood, and this makes them especially well equipped and prepared to be parents (Baran, 1989; ACLU, 1999). In my personal and clinical experience, and in these interviews, this was borne out. Every lesbian family that I encountered had given years of thought and preparation to their decision to have a child and most of these families *have* proven resilient and are thriving.

One important factor in successful families was each member's capacity to empathize with her partner thus allowing her to integrate her partner's needs with her own. Second, and closely related was her ability to identify with her partner's experience, enabling her to derive vicarious pleasure from her partner's relationship with their child, and thereby overcome feelings of envy, jealousy, or rejection. Third, was her ability to find and create positive parental identifications within herself. Difficulties developed as a result of an inability to draw upon these otherwise present capacities as a result of the force of regressive pulls induced by the parenting process.

It is the work, then, of therapy to help each individual recognize and address the various impediments that are interfering with her ability to create a viable and satisfying place for herself in the family. It is my hope that in clarifying some of the intrapsychic and relational dynamics which may be more or less particular to lesbian families, that these couples and the therapists working with them will be better prepared to navigate these issues effectively. And, if we agree with Tolstoy, that all happy families are alike, while unhappy families are different, then it is as much the case for lesbian families as for any other.

NOTES

1. For purposes of focus, this paper refers only to lesbian couples who choose to have children together. This is not meant to overlook lesbian step-families, single lesbian mothers, or gay fathers, all of whom share many of these issues, as well as ones deriving from their own unique circumstances. Likewise, for purposes of brevity, I will use the term *family* to refer to parents and child(ren). This in no way is intended to imply that couples without children are not families in themselves.

2. Centerkids is a New York City based organization offering services and support to gay and lesbian families.

3. Three African-American, three Latina, two Asian,

4. Certainly there are couples who have resolved their difference by not having children, but these were not part of my sample

5. I will be discussing dyadic and triadic issues in a later section of this paper.

6. It would be wrong to attribute the desire not to have a child solely to unresolved early conflicts. Schwartz (1998) reminds us that women may choose to be childfree yet express their generativity in a variety ways. Historically, lesbians were forced to do so since parenthood was largely denied them. Now that the option to parent is more possible there is often pressure on lesbians, as there has always been on heterosexual women, to have babies.

7. In fact, it is not always so easy to become pregnant

8. Adoptive couples rarely expressed this concern about the primary adoptive mother.

9. It might be expected that an individual with strong dyadic needs will choose to become involved with someone with comparable needs.

10. I wish to emphasize here that dyadic problems are not unique to lesbian families. They are also seen in heterosexual couples where the mother becomes overly involved with the children and the father finds himself on the periphery of the family. Again, social constructs may allow the father to organize this situation in such a way as to tolerate it, although it results in greater distance in the couple. However, it does also lead to marital failure, particularly if the husband is unable or unwilling to be relegated to the sidelines.

REFERENCES

Abelin, E.L. (1980). Triangulation, the role of the father and the origins of core gender identity during the rapprochement subphase. In *Rapprochement*, R. Lax, S. Bach, & J. Burland (eds). New York: Aronson, pp. 151-169

ACLU Fact Sheet: Overview of Lesbian and Gay Parenting, Adoption and Foster Care, April 6, 1999.

Baran, A. and Pannor, R. (1989). *Lethal secrets: Parents: the shocking consequences and unsolved problems of artificial insemination*. New York: Warner Books.

Benedek, T. (1959). Parenthood as a developmental phase: a contribution to libido theory, *Journal of the American Psychoanalytic Association*, 7:389-417.

Blos, P., Jr. 1985. Intergenerational separation-individuation: Treating the mother-infant pair. *Psychoanalytic study of the child*, 40:41-50.

Butler, J. (1995). Melancholy gender-refused identifications. *Psychoanalytic Dialogues*, 5(2); 165-180

Crawford, S. (1987). Lesbian families: psychosocial stress and the family-building process. In Boston Lesbian Psychology Collective (eds.) *Lesbian Psychologies*. Chicago: University of Illinois Press. pp. 195-214.

Crespi, L. (1997). From baby boom to gayby boom: Twenty-five years of psychoanalysis in the lesbian community. In Kiersky, S. and Gould, E. (eds.) *Moving violations: lesbians, psychoanalysis and culture*. New York: International Universities (in Press).

Frankfeldt, V.R.L. (1999). Maternal conflicts activated by the child's separation-individuation: a maturational opportunity. Unpublished manuscript.

Glazer, D. (1998). Lesbian mothers: a foot in two worlds, *Psychoanalysis and Psychotherapy*, 16(1), 145-151.

Kotelchuck, M. (1976). The infant's relationship to the father in *The role of the father in child development*, M.E. Lamb (ed). New York: Wiley, pp 329-344.

Mahler, M., Bergman A., & Pine, F. (1967). *The psychological birth of the human infant*. New York: Basic Books.

Pruet, K.D. (1983). Infants of primary nurturing fathers in *Psychoanalytic Study of the Child*, 38:257-276.

Schwartz, A.E. (1998). *Sexual subjects: Lesbians, gender and psychoanalysis*. New York: Routledge.

Tasker, F. and Golombok, S. (1997). *Growing up in a lesbian family: Effects on child development*. New York, Guilford Press.

Tolstoy, L. 1875 *Anna Karenina* Chap 1, p. 1.

Winnicott, D.W. (1956). Primary maternal preoccupation. In *Collected papers: Through pediatrics to psychoanalysis*. New York: Basic Books, pp. 300-305 (1958).

Lesbian Motherhood:
Restorative Choice
or Developmental Imperative?

Deborah F. Glazer, PhD

SUMMARY. Motherhood is a developmental phase that offers enhanced opportunities for intrapsychic growth and restoration. The idea of restorative motherhood may have special relevance for some women who have grown up to have a primary lesbian self identification. However, it must be recognized that the intrapsychic importance of a developmental option does not make that choice a developmental imperative. *[Article copies available for a fee from The Haworth Document Delivery Service: 1-800-342-9678. E-mail address: <getinfo@haworthpressinc.com> Website: <http://www.HaworthPress.com> © 2001 by The Haworth Press, Inc. All rights reserved.]*

KEYWORDS. Lesbian, motherhood, development, generativity, gender, childlessness, fertility, pregnancy

The psychoanalytic understanding of the intrapsychic role of motherhood has changed significantly since Freud's (1925) early understanding of the wish for a baby as a compensatory structure aimed at warding off a woman's recognition of her own castration. As early as the 1940s, theorists such as Deutsch (1945) saw the wish to mother as a complex developmental outcome. Rather than being a single, linear

---

Dr. Deborah F. Glazer is Supervisor and Faculty Member, Psychoanalytic Institute, The Postgraduate Center for Mental Health.

Address correspondence to: Deborah F. Glazer, PhD, 425 West 23 Street, Suite 1A, New York, NY 10011 (E-mail: dfglazer@aol.com).

[Haworth co-indexing entry note]: "Lesbian Motherhood: Restorative Choice or Developmental Imperative?" Glazer, Deborah F. Co-published simultaneously in *Journal of Gay & Lesbian Psychotherapy* (The Haworth Medical Press, an imprint of The Haworth Press, Inc.) Vol. 4, No. 3/4, 2001, pp. 31-43; and: *Gay and Lesbian Parenting* (ed: Deborah F. Glazer, and Jack Drescher) The Haworth Medical Press, an imprint of The Haworth Press, Inc., 2001, pp. 31-43. Single or multiple copies of this article are available from The Haworth Document Delivery Service [1-800-342-9678, 9:00 a.m. - 5:00 p.m. (EST). E-mail address: getinfo@haworthpressinc.com].

defensive development, she believed that the motherhood was a genuine developmental goal comprised of a complex interaction of multiple intrapsychic longings and wishes. She even believed that the wish to mother was not a singular goal, but that was reflected in multiple strivings, such as the wish to be pregnant, the wish to nurture, etc.

Today's psychoanalytic theorists and postmodern thinkers (D'Ercole, 1996) are questioning the concept that the intrapsychic world and the subjective experience of the self are concretely set in place by early to middle childhood. Rather, these theorists teach us to view the self as ever growing and changing, reconstructing components of identity throughout life in response to internal and external experiences and relationships. If the experience of the self is a living breathing, oscillating experience, as opposed to the fixed and rigid construct developed in early childhood as is previously understood by psychoanalysis, it will, as Erikson (1950) originally postulated, be amenable to change throughout the passages of adult life, not just during childhood. That would include the powerful intrapsychic growth brought about through procreation and parenting. Erikson writes that the

> fashionable insistence on dramatizing the dependence of children on adults often blinds us to the dependence of the older generation to the younger one. (p. 266)

In her 1959 paper entitled "Parenthood as a Developmental Phase," Therese Benedek discussed the developmental, restorative aspects of parenting. According to Benedek

> personality development continues beyond adolescence, under the influence of reproductive physiology and that parenthood utilizes the same primary processes which operate from infancy on in mental growth and development. (p. 389)

Benedek believes that there are "reciprocal ego developments" (p. 393) in both mother and child, which afford the mother the opportunity for a regressive experience that allows for the reworking of numerous childhood developmental themes. In discussing the regressive fantasies reactivated in pregnancy and early motherhood, Mendell (1998) suggests that the denial of the intrapsychic changes evoked by motherhood is due precisely to the nature of maternal fantasies and the subsequent intrapsychic changes. She notes that

> psychoanalytic opinion is divided about the normality of these experiences, both because that concept of continued intrapsychic

development, not just reworking of older conflicts is relatively recent and not generally accepted, but because the type of primitive regressive experiences which mothers have seems too similar to pathological states. (p. 107)

The aforementioned authors discuss parenting as evoking the reworking numerous childhood themes including: narcissistic issues; themes of confidence/an inner sense of "goodness; merger/individuation; and omnipotence."

MOTHERING AND A LESBIAN IDENTITY

In addition to these general developmental concepts issues related to motherhood may have special relevance for some women who have grown up to have a primary lesbian self identification. In recent years, much has been written about the unique developmental passages and experiences faced by many gay men and lesbians as a result of growing up gay in a heterosexist environment. One area of much speculation relates to the interplay of gender and sexual orientation. As Magee and Miller (1997) note:

In many psychoanalytic discussions homosexuality is prima facie example of gender identity disturbance. . . . Lesbian women are thought to have too much identification with their fathers, too little identification with their mothers, or both. (p. 179)

They suggest that gender is not a fixed attribute, like physical anatomy. Instead, gender is something learned, proscribed by the culture. They suggest that the way a woman experiences her self and her gender is continually reassessed and reevaluated during her life span. They also note that "[f]ailures or refusals to make expected gender presentations disturb the social landscape, upset the social order" (p. 180).

Representations of gender that are not in keeping with societal norms create powerful feelings of anxiety. These anxieties can be experienced by the others dealing with a gender "refusenik" (Schwartz, 1998), but more importantly for the purposes of this paper, they can be experienced as powerful feelings of anxiety and inadequacy within the "refusenik" herself. In other words, same sex desire can lead an individual to feel that there are less adequate representations of their gender than their heterosexual counterparts. Butler (1995) discusses the concept that lesbians and gay men may often experience a sense of being "monstrous" as a result of their same sex desire when gender, as we societally define it, is based on a heterosexual paradigm. According to Butler, gender, as we define it, evolves out of a recognition of heterosexual desire and a repudiation of same sex desire. The individual who experiences powerful or primary same sex desire experiences herself as not quite woman, but not quite man, and, therefore, inadequate, if not monstrous, in both realms.

In a 1998 paper entitled "The Body as Battleground: Same Sex Desire and the Gendered Self," I wrote that

> many of my patients enter treatment organizing their self experience around themes of gender and sexual orientation. These organizing self identifications interact in ways that can result in themes and symptoms that need to be addressed in the analytic work . . . recognition of one's same sex desire and homosexual object choice can result in feelings of alienation from one's body. Symptoms exhibited by these patients include: sexual inhibitions, feelings of shame or inadequacy in their bodies, substance abuse, obesity, and psychic numbing.

I suspect that part of the heterosexual standard of gender and bodily adequacy by which people measure themselves is the capacity to parent. In the play that I have observed in children, the identification as "mommy" or "daddy" seems to precede a recognition of erotic love or heterosexual union.

Notman and Lester (1988) believe that the recognition of her ability to procreate is an formative component in a woman's self esteem. They write that

> [f]or a woman, knowing that she is capable of bearing children has been critical in the development of her sense of femininity, gender identity, and self-esteem, even if as an adult she chooses not to actually have children. The awareness of her reproductive potential is part of her self-image. (p. 139)

They go on to note that for many women, an important "element of the procreative wish is . . . to be an adult like the parents" (p. 142).

Some lesbians may find the development of the ability to view themselves as "grown-up women" may be somewhat complicated. For many women, both lesbian and heterosexual, passage through the adults stages of life can involve an increased identification with mother. In fact, it seems that the tightrope between identification with mother and the individuation from mother is a lifelong process that can come to the forefront at different periods in a woman's life. Mendell (op. cit.) notes that pregnancy and the experiences of mothering can reactivate the "one body fantasy" across the three generations of grandmother, mother, and baby. Joan Larkin (1997) describes this in her poem "Legacy."

> When my mother finally left her body/it was mine to keep/along with her ring,/some blackened silver,/a box of Jewish books./At first I thought it would be a difficult fit/but here a tuck and a seam there let out/and you'd swear it was made for me/. . . Sunday I'll walk down the aisle at my daughter's wedding/and the thin breasts in grey silk/will be my mother's. (p. 41)

Lesbians may face even greater difficulty as they navigate the intricacies of identification and individuation as various life passages evoke the identification with mother while at the same time consolidating a sexual identification that is often significantly different from mother.

The idea of experiencing the self as "adult" like the parent can hold special meaning for some lesbians as they are often excluded from many of the socially sanctioned rituals signifying the move from child to adult. This can be exacerbated by certain theoretical and societal biases which have resulted in some lesbians fearing that their same sex choice erotic object choice leaves them immature, not fully "grown-up." This is in keeping with traditional psychoanalytic theories of lesbianism as regressive sexuality that have pervaded our culture, and can be seen in the writings of cultural critics like Camille Paglia (1990). According to Paglia, the values of western culture dictate that the further one has moved away from mother, the more intellectually and emotionally evolved one is. As a romantic relationship with another woman can superficially mirror the relationship with mother, and may even reawaken old maternal conflicts, some women may fear that they can never fully grow up while being in a lesbian relationship. These fears can be exacerbated by the previously discussed fears of not being "adequately" woman. The recognition that one can be in love with a woman and still mother can counteract some of those fears, and can consolidate and validate the move from dependent to care giver.

In addition, all developmental outcomes require mourning for those paths and objects relinquished (Fast, 1979). Crespi (1995) writes that part of the development of a positive lesbian identity requires a mourning of societal status and privilege, as well as a mourning of the ego ideals, of the expected heterosexual developmental outcome. The presumption of heterosexuality with which we are all raised may exacerbate the sense of loss and mourning associated with the recognition of a primarily lesbian erotic life. Crespi notes that lesbians must mourn the ability to create a child with their loved one. Much of the mourning experienced in the coming out process may be the mourning of that capacity to parent, in general, as the development of a gay identification has traditionally foreclosed the possibility of parenting for many women. Despite all of the advances in gay and lesbian rights, and the "gayby boom" of recent years, the headlines are still full of children who have been taken from their gay or lesbian parents due to court's rulings of parental inadequacy due to sexual orientation.

Schwartz (op. cit.) notes that some lesbians experience feelings of grief and emptiness resulting from their inability to mother. While recognizing that there is often an overreliance and overidealization of mothering as the only, or most adequate, form of generativity, she writes that

> [c]hildfree lesbians often express a deep sense of loss or projected impoverishment when they foresee a life foreclosed from the possibilities of transcending more immediate narcissistic interests through generative participation in the broader culture. (p. 95)

For some women, the capacity to mother also may facilitate the coming out process, as there are now fewer losses to mourn in relinquishing the presumed heterosexual outcome. For many lesbians that I have seen in treatment, the recent increase in the awareness that they can parent provides a sense of citizenship in the larger culture that had been foreclosed to prior generations.

RESTORATIVE MOTHERING

In addition to the intrapsychic issues related to identity, some women who grow up to be lesbian experience early familial/interpersonal difficulties related to their representation of gender and their early expressions of desire. Kiersky (1998) writes for some lesbians, the early family life, particularly regarding states of desire, involves in a lack of parental mirroring and recognition that yields feelings of inauthenticity She evokes the image of the velveteen rabbit, who is made real through love, as representative of this dilemma. However, while Kiersky discusses the love of the parent (or later, perhaps, the analyst) as the source of feelings of authenticity, the fairy tale implies that it is the love of a child that makes one real.

For some women the experience of mothering, being loved by a child, and making a family through connection to a child can be particularly healing and validating. In an autobiographical account of her experiences as a lesbian mother, Dorothy Allison (1999) writes

> Family means two different things to me. One is the family of my birth. It's my nation. The people I trust and understand even when I don't trust them for a minute. "Family" is a big word, but very painful. The word "family" hides everything–including the people that you are despised by yet hold on to, and the people to whom you do not want to give your address. (p. 17)

But, Allison goes on to note that creating a family within the gay and lesbian community, and creating a family with her lover, their son, the donor, and grandparents has caused her to reevaluate the word "family," and to experience a sense of love, safety, and connectedness that she could not feel within her family of origin. Thus, it appear that for some women, the experiences of mothering in later life can have healing or restorative effects related to feelings of interpersonal connectedness and authenticity.

The following clinical vignettes are examples of ways in which the psychological growth worked toward in treatment was facilitated and consolidated by the experience of mothering. Dana entered treatment presenting a complex, multiply determined clinical picture. Her presenting problem was a powerful sexual inhibition, that left her unable to be sexually active with her female lover of numerous years. As treatment progressed, it became evident that Dana had been raised by a depressed and depleted mother who had, herself, been raised in a neglectful, violently abusive home. Both of Dana's parents were alcohol abusers. Dana reluctantly began to report numerous incidents of feeling ignored or overwhelmed by the chaos in her home. As the work ensued, more symptoms came to light. Dana was bulimic, and had a deeply troubled relationship with her body. She felt shamed and embarrassed of her appetites, and was fearful and conflicted about gratifying any of them. While she was harshly self-critical of her sexual desires, she also feared that her lesbianism was symptomatic of emotional and sexual immaturity. She fantasized about having sexual relations with a man to prove her passage into womanhood. Dana had always worked as a nanny, taking care of other women's children. This exacerbated her feeling of inadequacy as she viewed herself as capable of taking care of the babies of more powerfully feminine women, while believing her sexual development led her to be unable to mother.

As time passed, Dana became increasingly aware of her powerful wish to mother. This required working through some significant issues. Dana had to mourn the idea of conceiving through sexual intercourse, as she and her lover opted to use an unknown donor. She had to allow herself to acknowledge and accept her appetites, so that she could sufficiently nourish her body to allow for conception and a healthy pregnancy. Despite her fantasies that her body was inadequately female, Dana conceived on her first attempt, which became a source of great pride. Rather than battle the roundness of the womanliness that Dana felt undeserving of and threatened by, she took great pride in the blossoming of her breasts and abdomen. Throughout the pregnancy, Dana was filled with fears that her body was not a sufficient environment in which a baby could grow, which could be seen as an identification with the depleted mother. When she gave birth to a healthy child, she took pride in her ability to nurse and care for him. This could be understood as Dana's ability to revel in the cornucopia fantasy (Mendell, ibid.), where Dana was able to both become and become reunited with the "ever flowing breast" (p. 92). The experience of mothering allowed Dana to find a way to identify with some aspects of mother, by allowing herself the right to those things "women" can have. At the same time, it allowed for a disidentification/separation, as she saw that she did not have to be the type of woman/mother that her mother had become by becoming sexually active or procreating.

Laura entered treatment at the request of her lover of many years, who complained about Laura's emotional distance and the difficulty she had in committing to the relationship. Laura's lover had a middle childhood aged daughter, and wished for the threesome to live together as a family. Laura was unable to entertain the idea. While Laura had been out since college, and had been active in lesbian sexual politics, it became clear that she felt like a misfit in the world at large. She felt shamed about her bodily representation. She experienced herself as a hybrid that could only feel at home in exclusively lesbian settings. Laura described her mother as an emotionally disturbed woman. For Laura, the idea of growing up to be like her mother was intolerable, and she had numerous childhood fantasies/wishes of growing up to be a man (which is not to be confused with transsexualism). The passages of adolescence were difficult for Laura, as she could not engage in the boy-girl rituals. By adult life, Laura had become somewhat isolated. She had a number of friends, but could not allow herself access to romantic intimacy or family.

As treatment progressed, Laura worked toward allowing herself to become more involved with her lover and daughter. She allowed herself access to those aspects of herself that she had warded off, in a disidentification with mother, and that she felt unworthy of, as a sexual hybrid. She was also able to finally grieve the feeling of being inadequately nurtured. This allowed Laura to become involved in a pattern of giving and receiving nurturance and love that had been lost in her childhood. She began to experience herself as more of a valid citizen of the world. Her connectedness and joy were represented in a Mother's Day card she received during her last year of treatment, which was addressed "To my co-mother" and signed by her "co-daughter."

MOTHERING: CHOICE NOT IMPERATIVE

It is important to note that "achieving" motherhood is not an essential step in adult development, and it is not the only way to achieve generativity. In addition, an over reliance of the concept of mothering as healing can involve magical thinking that can have some problematic outcomes. It is not uncommon for women to have children with the anticipation of feeling whole or healed, only to find that after the initial joys of pregnancy and motherhood, they have intrapsychically returned to the same place they began. In addition, they have the added stress of having to care for a baby who has disappointed them by not causing the sense of healing and connectedness which they had expected. As Benedeck (op. cit.) points out, failures or disappointments in the symbiotic union of the mother/child relationship can "induce a regression in the mother that intensifies the regressive components of her receptive needs" (p. 396). Thus, the mothering experience, which was partly motivated by a wish to resolve ambivalent feelings about the experience of the self and the relationships with early objects can actually intensify the dependency needs, serving to exacerbate feelings of depression and aggression.

The following vignette offers an example of a situation where magical wishes related to the healing powers of pregnancy and mothering lead to anger and disappointment which could lead to increased psychological and interpersonal difficulty. Jane and Sue are a lesbian couple with a 3 year old, who entered treatment complaining that they could not agree upon whether to have a second child. Sue, their child's biological mother, expressed feelings of desperation for a second child, while Jane was concerned that she would be overwhelmed by the demands of taking care of yet another person. Sue described that her pregnancy filled her with joy, and that she experienced powerful feelings of pride and completeness in the early mothering experience. However, as time passed, Sue began to experience a resurgence of her feelings of loss and isolation that were rooted in her own childhood experience. She stated that she could never be complete without another child, and that their first child could never be complete without a sibling. Powerful feelings of rage at having her needs thwarted were evoked by her lover's resistance to go ahead with Sue's second pregnancy. Sue's belief that she can be healed by a second child may ultimately lead to the destruction of the family that she already has.

The experiences of mothering in a lesbian couple can also have its own particular stresses. Sharing mothering with a female partner can, for some, evoke complicated feelings of competition and a reawakening of stressful Oedipal themes. It increases the need to publicly "come-out," and can reawaken fears of homophobia (Glazer, 1998).

In recent years, in the lesbian community, women are feeling pressures to mother that are beginning to approximate the pressures for heterosexual women. At this point, it seems important to differentiate the importance of the recognition of the capacity to parent with the imperative to parent. While procreative activity can yield intrapsychic growth and development, mothering is certainly not the only way to reach "maturity," "femininity," or "generativity." Erikson (op. cit.) notes that generativity is not solely the issue of parents giving to children. Rather, it has shaped our society in numerous way, making "man the teaching and instituting as well as learning animal" (p. 266). He notes that there are "individuals who, through misfortune or through special and genuine gifts in other directions, do not apply this drive to their own offspring" (p. 267). And notes that generativity can be fully gratified through other forms of productivity or creativity.

Similarly, when Notman and Lester (op. cit.) write of the importance of the awareness of her reproductive potential in the development of a woman's sense of adequacy, they stress that is the recognition of that capacity, as opposed to the fulfillment of that capacity, that affects the self-esteem. They write that "[h]aving a baby although a pivotal event psychologically and physically, may not provide the only path to attain adult status as a women" (p. 139), and recommend that psychoanalytic research needs to explore other pathways in adult developmental that do not include parenting.

As Lesser (1991) notes, it is not the decision to mother that results in a sense of intrapsychic well-being. Nor is it the decision not to mother that results in feelings of grief and mourning. Rather, it is the belief that the path to mothering was foreclosed against one's wishes as a result of external forces. She conducted a study interviewing lesbians who had decided not to have children. She determined that

> [w]omen who feel that they have made the choice not to have children seemed to feel the least regrets. although they had to work through feelings of sadness and loss, it was in a context of knowing that they could have chosen to have children and that they decided against it by weighing all the possibilities. Women who felt that they couldn't have children because of circumstances beyond their control (e.g., not having a partner or financial stability), seemed to be the most ambivalent. (p. 90)

As Schwartz (op cit) mentions, for a number of lesbians there is the belief that their lesbianism has foreclosed the road to motherhood. For these women, the decision not to mother may be more conflicted.

CONCLUSION

As we look at the fluidity of the intrapsychic world throughout the life span, it becomes increasingly important to question how the stages and experiences of adult life affect the inner world. Mothering has always been an important life passage for women, and increased rights and technologies are making this an increasingly prevalent experience for lesbians. While mothering can have significant developmental and restorative features, it is important to recognize that motherhood is an option, not a developmental imperative.

REFERENCES

Allison, D. (1999). The Allison/Layman Family. *Love Makes a Family: Portraits of Lesbian, Gay, Bisexual, and Transgender Parents and Their Families.* Kaeser, G, Gillespie, P. and Weston, K. (eds). University of Massachussets Press, Amherst, Mass.

Benedek, T. (1959). Parenthood as a developmental phase: A contribution to libido theory. *Journal of the American Psychoanalytic Association*, 2:389-417.

Butler, Judith (1995). Melancholy gender–refused identification. *Pscychoanalytic Dialogues*, 5: 165-180.

Crespi, Lee (1995). Some thought on the role of mourning in the development of a positive lesbian identity. *Disorienting Sexuality: Psychoanalytic Reappraisals of Sexual Identies.* Deminici, T. & Lesser, R. eds., Routledge, NY.

D'Ercole, Ann (1996). Postmodern ideas about gender and sexuality: The lesbian woman redundancy. *Psychoanalysis and Psychotherapy*, 13: 142-152.

Deutsch, Helene (1945). *Psychology of Women: Vol. II.* Grune & Strutton, N.Y.

Erikson, E. (1950). *Childhood and Society.* W.W. Norton, NY (1963).

Freud, S. (1931). Female sexuality. *Standard Edition*, 21: 221-243, Hogarth Press, London.

Fast, Irene (1979). Developments in gender identity: Gender differentiation in girls. *International Journal of Psychoanalysis*, 60: 443-453.

Glazer, D. (1998). Lesbian mothers: A foot in two worlds. *Psychoanalysis and Psychotherapy*, 16: 145-151.

_____ (1998). The body as battle ground: Same sex desire and the gendered self. Paper presented at the International Federation of Psychoanalytic Education, Fordham University, New York.

Kiersky, Sandra (1996). Exiled desire: The problem of reality in psychoanalysis and lesbian experience. *Psychoanalysis and Psychotherapy*, 13: 130-141.

Larkin, J. (1997). *Cold River.* Painted Leaf Press.

Lesser, R. (1991). Deciding not to become a mother. *Lesbians at Midlife: The Creative Transition.* Sang, B., Warshow, J. and Smith, A., eds, Spinsters Book Co., San Francisco, CA.

Magee, M. and Miller, D. (1997). *Lesbian Lives: Psychoanalytic Narratives Old & New*. The Analytic Press, NJ.

Mendell, D. (1998). An exploration of three typical maternal fantasies: The cornucopia fantasy, the fantasy of parthenogeneisi, and the one-body fantasy. *Psychoanalysis and Psychotherapy*, 16: 85-110.

Notman, Malkah T. and Lester, Eva (1988). Pregnancy: Theoretical considerations. *Psychoanalytic Inquiry*, 8: 139-169.

Paglia, C. (1990). *Sexual personae: Art and Decadence from Nefertiti to Emily Dickinson*. Yale University Press, London & New Haven.

Schwartz, A. (1998). *Sexual Subjects: Lesbians, Gender, and Psychoanalysis*. Routledge, New York.

Inevitable Disclosure:
Countertransference Dilemmas
and the Pregnant Lesbian Therapist

Sandra Silverman, CSW

SUMMARY. When the therapist is pregnant her personal life enters the treatment room. This can present a dilemma for the pregnant lesbian therapist who may feel that it is impossible to respond to the patient's questions without disclosing her sexual orientation. The author asserts that in order for the work to progress in an authentic, open, and spontaneous manner, the therapist must not feel that she is hiding a significant part of herself from her patients. Issues such as disclosure, enactment, use of countertransference and the subjectivity of the therapist are addressed. *[Article copies available for a fee from The Haworth Document Delivery Service: 1-800-342-9678. E-mail address: <getinfo@haworthpressinc.com> Website: <http://www.HaworthPress.com> © 2001 by The Haworth Press, Inc. All rights reserved.]*

KEYWORDS. Countertransference, transference, pregnant, analyst, disclosure, lesbian, sexual orientation, enactment, relational psychoanalysis

---

Sandra Silverman is Supervisor, Institute for Contemporary Psychotherapy; and Faculty Member and Supervisor, Psychoanalytic Psychotherapy Study Center. The author also maintains a private practice in Manhattan.

Address correspondence to: Sandra Silverman, CSW, 153 Waverly Place, Suite 10E, New York, NY 10014 (E-mail: Sgsilverman@aol.com).

[Haworth co-indexing entry note]: "Inevitable Disclosure: Countertransference Dilemmas and the Pregnant Lesbian Therapist." Silverman, Sandra. Co-published simultaneously in *Journal of Gay & Lesbian Psychotherapy* (The Haworth Medical Press, an imprint of The Haworth Press, Inc.) Vol. 4, No. 3/4, 2001, pp. 45-61; and: *Gay and Lesbian Parenting* (ed: Deborah F. Glazer, and Jack Drescher) The Haworth Medical Press, an imprint of The Haworth Press, Inc., 2001, pp. 45-61. Single or multiple copies of this article are available from The Haworth Document Delivery Service [1-800-342-9678, 9:00 a.m. - 5:00 p.m. (EST). E-mail address: getinfo@haworthpressinc.com].

The pregnancy of the therapist is undeniable proof of the therapist's heterosexuality.

Fenster, Phillips & Rapoport, *The Therapist's Pregnancy*

A patient I have been seeing for several years walks into a session.
She hesitates for a moment and then begins, "I've been wondering
about something. Are you pregnant?" I confirm for her that I am and
she congratulates me. As the patient elaborates on her thoughts and
feelings about my pregnancy I realize that she has taken it as a definite
indication that I, like her, am heterosexual. I find myself becoming
anxious and uncomfortable. The assumption that a pregnant woman is
involved with a man is not unusual and so I can't attribute it all to
transference. I feel as if my silence is leading my patient to an erro-
neous belief. I am unsure how to proceed. A sudden disclosure that I
am a lesbian does not feel like an appropriate course of action. However, not saying anything at all makes me feel increasingly uneasy.

When I was pregnant, most of my patients asked me about my
personal life. These questions made me acutely aware of my sexual
orientation and of the possible consequences of disclosing it. Patients
who were not aware of my sexual orientation generally considered my
pregnancy as evidence of my heterosexuality. This felt strange to me. I
felt I was misleading my own patients with whom I had worked to
develop a trusting relationship. Now, having learned of my pregnancy,
they had the sense that they knew more about me but part of what they
felt they now knew, and felt that I had told them, was inaccurate. These
"assumptions" can be considered transference but they are certainly
not transference distortions. In the world as we know it, to be pregnant
is to be heterosexual. Perhaps there will be a time when sexual orientation is not assumed and people will not be certain of heterosexuality
based on pregnancy and parenthood but we have not arrived there yet.
To act as if we have is a denial of the reality of our time.

In my work with patients during my pregnancy I often felt I was not
being emotionally honest or available to them. I felt constrained, as if
I was hiding a part of myself from them. They had spoken of my
personal life and made assumptions about it, assumptions that I could
not entirely consider transference and that had powerful personal and
cultural meaning for me. I was unsure of how much to disclose and
how much to keep private.

When the pregnant therapist is a lesbian decisions about self-disclosure are complicated in a different way than for the therapist who is heterosexual. I was concerned that my patients would reject or devalue me if they knew of my sexual orientation. I recognize that these were my personal countertransferential feelings however I believe that the psychoanalytic community's historically negative views of homosexuality (Drescher, 1995), and of disclosing it to one's patients, contributed to my countertransferential concern. This left me with the feeling that I was hiding a significant part of myself from my patients. There is a difference between hiding and choosing not to disclose. If the therapist is hiding, her affect will be inhibited, causing distance between herself and her patient and limiting the depth of the work. Not to hide does not necessarily mean coming out to your patients. It simply means that the analyst feels comfortable enough with the *possibility* of becoming known that she is able to be emotionally and affectively present in her work with her patient. Whether I disclosed my sexual orientation or not, it quickly became clear to me that my pregnancy had brought my personal life into the treatment room and my feelings about it were affecting the work.

Pregnancy is a time of physical and emotional vulnerability. The increased exposure that it brings can cause considerable anxiety in the pregnant therapist (Fenster, Phillips, Rapoport, 1986). When the therapist is pregnant her personal life, and this includes her sexual life, is suddenly in the room with her and her patient. Therapists tend to disclose more to their patients during their pregnancy than at other times and even those who prefer to remain anonymous to their patients find it impossible to do so when they are pregnant (Fenster et al., 1986). The visibility of their pregnancy is a personal disclosure in and of itself, significantly changing the atmosphere in the treatment room.

When the therapist is pregnant the work becomes more complicated because when she explores her patient's feelings about her pregnancy she is also asking the patient to examine his or her feelings about what the therapist may be experiencing. And, as Aron (1996) has written on self-disclosure and the subjectivity of the analyst,

> By focusing on the patient's experience of the analyst's subjectivity, you are likely to stir up conflicts in both the patient and yourself about knowing and being known. It is one thing to not reveal much to your patient when you have not focused the analytic lens on this area of inquiry, but, once you do, the patient may be unable to tolerate not receiving any response, and it may

feel torturous to you to not provide some response . . . Included in what patients know about their analysts, but that they may not know that they know, is their recognition of the therapist's conflicts about being known. (1986, p. 238)

For the pregnant therapist these include conflicts about the introduction of her personal life into the treatment relationship. How much will the patient ask? What will it feel like to have a major event in her personal life spoken about with her patients? How will the therapist's relational experience with her patient affect her decisions about how much to disclose? And, what experiences in the therapist's personal and professional life will inform her decision about how much to disclose to her patients?

Imber (1990) in her paper on the countertransference of the pregnant analyst writes, "The fantasies, wishes, conflicts and anxieties which being pregnant arouses, both personally and professionally, may result in denial and avoidance of highly charged material with patients." She points out that an awareness of countertransference, which is so essential to analytic work and which becomes considerably more complex during pregnancy, is often avoided by the pregnant analyst. If the analyst feels guilty that she is causing a disruption in the treatment she may become more defensive with regard to her countertransference reactions. In addition, concerns about her own physical health and feelings about the intrapsychic, interpersonal and familial changes that are occurring as she moves into the role of mother may prevent her from being open to the range of her countertransferential emotions.

Many of my feelings of misleading my patients with regard to my sexual orientation were related to my own life experience as a lesbian in our culture. In a discussion of lesbian coming out issues, Magee and Miller (1995) write about the confusion and deception that often occur in casual conversations.

The woman in a lesbian relationship who keeps silent is doing more than remaining private. At the very least she is keeping a secret; often the secret involves telling a lie. (p. 99)

This daily life reality carries over into the treatment room. The lesbian therapist's fear of the consequences of having her sexual orientation become known can make it difficult for her to determine one of the most critical aspects of self disclosure, that is, whether it opens up or forecloses the analytic work (Aron, 1996). Even if she has no intention of ever revealing her sexual orientation to her patient, the fear of becoming known as a lesbian and the anxiety about withholding this information can still have a significant impact on her work.

For the lesbian therapist who is pregnant, concerns about the social acceptance of her pregnancy add to her feelings of anxiety and vulnerability in her work with patients. The social experience of pregnancy is markedly different for a lesbian than it is for a heterosexual woman. The heterosexual woman who announces her pregnancy is typically received with joy, pride and excitement. For her, pregnancy is viewed as an accomplishment and it confirms her membership in heterosexual society. The pregnancy and parenthood of a lesbian is not socially or culturally sanctioned. The public response to it may be discomfort, confusion or disapproval, causing increased feelings of vulnerability in the pregnant woman who is a lesbian.

Pregnancy is psychically linked to heterosexual sex. Pines (1972) has described it as "a visible manifestation to the outside world that (the pregnant woman) has had a sexual relationship" (p. 334). Benedek (1973) notes that patients make various comments when they suspect that the therapist may be pregnant. These include comments about confidentiality, sexual concerns and statements that there is "something queer in the room" (Benedek, 1973). This being the case, the lesbian therapist is left with a dilemma: what does one do when there really is something, or rather someone, queer in the room?

How this dilemma might be handled is dependent upon whether the therapist has disclosed her sexual orientation to her patient and, upon the theoretical framework within which the therapist is working. Relational therapists view the analytic relationship as one in which both members are continuously affecting each other, even in the subtlest of ways. Within this two-person paradigm, an exploration of what transpires between patient and therapist is considered essential. It would be impossible for the therapist to remove herself and simply observe what is occurring in the treatment because her participation in the analytic relationship is continuous (Aron, 1996). The therapist will inevitably be pulled into enactments with the patient (Aron, 1996; Maroda, 1999; Mitchell, 1988; Renik, 1993). Understanding how and why these enactments occur is considered a crucial aspect of the work. In addition, countertransference disclosure is viewed as inevitable since we are always revealing ourselves to our patients in a variety of ways including silence and interpretation.

Maroda (1994, 1999) writes on the value of affective disclosure of countertransference and recognizes the exchange of genuine emotion between patient and therapist as central to therapeutic action. She notes the dangers of therapists inhibiting their affect, believing this contributes to therapist's acting out and impulsively revealing their countertransferential feelings at inopportune moments. The therapist's need for self-expression in such an intense relationship is, according to Maroda, "basic and inescapable" (p. 174). She writes,

> (M)ore damage is done when the analyst hides than when he or she is direct or honest. I believe that more harm is done to patients by well-meaning analysts, who do not want to 'burden' their patients than by honest, straightforward clinicians who admit to the realities of doing therapy. (p. 174)

If the therapist represses or denies her affect the patient is often left feeling confused and unsure of whether to trust her own perceptions. Maroda observes that when she is willing to be more open and risk taking with her patients, they are more willing to do so with her. She states that "the key to our success lies in our emotional availability and emotional honesty, not in our ability to remain above the fray" (1999, p. 182).

Some relational analysts have examined the concept of neutrality and questioned whether it is possible to take a neutral stance with regard to sexual orientation (Frommer, 1995; Blechner, 1993; Schwartz, 1993; Mitchell, 1997). Frommer (1995), in his paper on countertransference obscurity, discusses heterosexual therapists and their lack of countertransference awareness in working with gay patients. His thoughts can also be applied to gay or lesbian therapists working with patients of any sexual orientation. The neutral stance with regard to sexual orientation, according to Frommer,

> speaks more to what is apparent than real. At best it addresses the surface of the analytic encounter and is reductionistic and dangerous to the patient when the subtleties of the analyst's countertransference experience are not acknowledged and understood. (pp. 68-9)

For the gay or lesbian therapist, being homosexual in a heterosexual world makes it impossible not to have a wide range of intense countertransferential feelings when issues related to sexual orientation enter into the analytic relationship. These countertransferential feelings, especially if they involve shame or fear, may cause the therapist's affect to be inhibited. This may result in the therapist finding it difficult to be emotionally honest and available to her patients, leaving her with the feeling that she is hiding parts of herself from her patients rather than that she has made a clinically appropriate *choice* not to disclose. What follows are several case examples illustrating some of the counter-transference dilemmas I faced in my work and how I handled them during and after my pregnancy.

WORK WITH HETEROSEXUAL PATIENTS

Sarah

Many of these issues came up in my work with Sarah, a 30 year-old editor of children's books. She was in treatment with me for five years prior to my becoming pregnant. Having grown up with a mother who suffered from frequent, severe depressions and died when Sarah was seven years old, her life experience has been colored by loss. Sarah entered treatment hoping to address what she described as a "basic feeling of aloneness." She felt that this was probably a core aspect of her personality and perhaps therapy could help her learn to live with it. Despite having a number of close friendships and being well liked in both her professional and personal life, Sarah suffered from considerable feelings of loneliness and isolation. I found Sarah immediately engaging and enjoyed her quick, wry sense of humor. In our first session I noted an energetic, spunky quality in her. She said she often tried to subdue this part of herself as she felt it was indicative of self-centeredness and feared it would drive others away.

After her mother's death Sarah, an only child, remembers trying to keep her father's spirits up, working hard not to need too much from him. Sarah's family was devastated by the loss of Sarah's mother and dealt with this by rarely speaking about her. Her father remarried one year after Sarah's mother died and soon thereafter had two more children. The general attitude toward Sarah was that she was fortunate to get a new mother and a couple of younger siblings so soon after her mother's death. Sarah felt lost. She wondered about her mother, her depressions, and why she had died. She felt she was somehow responsible for this loss. Sarah's was a family that had always had many secrets and taught its members the importance of keeping things to oneself. Sarah learned to sense when someone was uncomfortable and not to ask questions of them. As a result, her fears and fantasies about her mother grew without any opportunity to talk with anyone about them.

I was aware of feeling protective and maternal towards Sarah from early on. She immersed herself in the treatment and there was a timeless and intimate feeling in the room. She saw me as a caring, consistent presence in her life. In the transference she expressed fears that her needs would devour me, that her dependence would make me want to get away from her and that her anger would be overwhelming for me. She preferred to think of me as not being real because then feelings of anger, disappointment, or attachment in either one of us would be less terrifying for her.

When I was six months pregnant Sarah walked into my office with a look of anticipation. She said she wanted to ask me something, "Are you pregnant?" I immediately answered, "Yes." I believe there was an unspoken awareness in both of us that we were talking in a way we never had before. She then began to speak about the thoughts she'd had prior to asking me whether or not I was pregnant. "You know, I didn't even know you were married," she said. I sat quietly and listened, or so I *thought*. Clearly, Sarah saw a reaction in me. She looked away, began to speak more about my pregnancy, stopped herself and then looked back at me and repeated, "It's just so strange because I didn't even know you were married." I felt increasingly uncomfortable. As much as I wanted to believe I was providing Sarah the space to continue talking about her feelings regarding my pregnancy, my countertransference was starting to fill the entire room. She said, in a reticent and confused way, "You are married aren't you?" I didn't know what to do. I felt unable to think. It didn't feel right to me to refuse to answer her question but I did not even know what the correct answer was. I blurted out, "Actually, I'm not married." "Oh!" she said, looking quite surprised. "Well," she continued, "marriage doesn't really mean that much," trying to rescue me, or perhaps both of us, from the awkwardness of the moment. As I regained my composure I asked Sarah how she felt about this new information. She made light of it and inquired about my due date and how much time I'd be taking off. She said she thought I'd make a great mother and spent the remainder of the session talking about a man she'd recently begun dating and her fears that the relationship did not have a future.

I felt completely baffled by what happened to me in that session. My interaction with Sarah was a perfect example of what Renik (1993) describes when he states that, "awareness of countertransference is always retrospective, preceded by countertransference enactment." I thought that I was prepared for what might arise with regard to my pregnancy but could not begin to know the extent and nature of my countertransferential feelings until they were enacted.

Why was I so overwhelmed? Why did I feel that I could not explore her question without answering it? Was I afraid she'd see me as defective and unable to help her if she knew I was not heterosexual? Would I be able to handle her negative feelings about my sexual orientation? Was I afraid of repeating the avoidance and denial that had gone on in her family? In that moment I lost sight of what my pregnancy might have meant to Sarah, and how it punctured the private and timeless feeling that she had experienced with me. All I could think about was whether answering her question would mean coming out to her. She was not asking me whether or not I was gay but I couldn't figure out how to answer her without giving her that information. On the other hand, refusing to answer seemed absurd. I'm the one who, via my pregnancy, brought my personal life into the treatment room. Telling her that I am not married only caused her more confusion. This session with Sarah brought to light my fears of what would happen if she found out about my sexual orientation.

In the following session I tried to explore Sarah's feelings about what had transpired between us. I acknowledged my discomfort and wondered how Sarah felt about it. She seemed equally uncomfortable with what had happened. In retrospect I feel that I did not push for too much exploration of the discomfort. I was still sorting out what had happened to me in the session and I was unsure how to keep my feelings of anxiety from overwhelming me once again. The more I sorted it through for myself and, over time, with Sarah, the freer I was able to be in my work with her. I believe that as I felt freer to express myself and my feelings, she felt freer to express her feelings about who I am to her.

Sarah said she thought there were a number of possible explanations for my not being married including that I was with a non-committal man or that I was gay. She focused primarily on the possibility that I was with a non-committal man, stating that this was the most frightening to her, as she feared it would be her own future. It was not until well after I returned from my leave that she began to discuss what it would mean for her if I were gay.

In the first year after my return from maternity leave our work focused primarily on Sarah's feelings of loss during and after my pregnancy. In the transference I had become the mother who abandoned her. She felt that she must not have been good enough for me to want to be with her. She must have been too flawed or too needy and so I had left her for my own child, about whom I truly cared. She wondered if she had "glue," by which she meant the ability to form an attachment with others and not lose them. Sarah spoke about the loss of her mother in a new way. She now felt that no one could be the mother she did not have and saw her self as truly motherless. A deeper mourning process ensued. As we worked through her feelings about my pregnancy, which included anger, disappointment and hurt, new questions emerged about who I am outside of our sessions and what our relationship is to one another.

Sarah returned to the question of whether or not I am a lesbian. She said that because she has a number of lesbian friends, she was surprised at how uncomfortable she found the thought of my being gay. In her maternal transference to me I had been the *heterosexual* mother who she could look up to and admire. If I am a lesbian then Sarah was not sure if she could look up to me in the same way. She feared that if we were different in this way then I could not feel as close to her as she had thought. What was more difficult for her to talk about was how hard it would be for her to feel close to me if I am a lesbian. How could she identify with me if I am a lesbian and she is heterosexual? My lesbian identity would be a profound disappointment to Sarah and an indication that I am flawed and imperfect.

I believe the enactment that occurred in my work with Sarah during my pregnancy resulted from her fear of seeing that I am not who she wants me to be, as well as from my feelings of vulnerability connected with the pregnancy itself and, with my anxiety about the potential disclosure of my sexual orientation. My own fears of how my child would feel about having a mother who is a lesbian also played a role in my resistance to exploring more deeply what it would mean for Sarah to have a therapist who is a lesbian. Imber (1990) notes that it was only after her maternity leave, with a lessening of her sense of vulnerability, that she was able to more fully explore some of the issues that arose for her patients during her pregnancy. I have found this to be true for myself as well. I attribute it not only to my decreasing feelings of the vulnerability associated with pregnancy, but also to my increased comfort and security in the role of lesbian mother. Although Sarah still does not want to know, definitively, whether or not I am a lesbian, and I have not told her, we are now able to talk about it as a real possibility. Recently she has spoken about how scary and painful it is for her to think that I might be gay. I have felt sad for her as she experiences the inevitable disappointment that I am not everything she wants me to be. I believe it is only with this exploration that Sarah will be able to know me, or anyone else, as human rather than perfect. While this is still difficult terrain, I no longer feel the same fear of what would happen if Sarah did find out that I am gay as I did in the session in which she inquired about my "marriage." As a result, I am able to be more emotionally present in the treatment and our work has deepened considerably.

Jamie

Unlike Sarah who asked me directly about my personal life, Jamie, a 26 year old heterosexual woman, learned about my life through revelations I was not even aware I had made. When we make deliberate revelations to our patients we experience a sense of control over our work. However, much of what we reveal to our patients is revealed inadvertently. Frank (1997) writes that "By definition, *inadvertent* revelations are unplanned. They are not part of formal technique–that aspect of the analyst's participation that can be to a significant degree conscious, controlled and deliberate" (p. 287). In my work with Jamie, I realized not just how much I may have communicated inadvertently, but also how much I had colluded with her in not talking about what may have been known, including my sexual orientation.

One day I ran into Jamie, who I'd been working with for three years, when I was with my partner, our toddler son (born to my partner), and our newborn daughter. At the following session she commented, "Gee, you have everything that I'm hoping to have. You've just got it with a woman instead of a man." When I told her that I was not aware that she knew I was in a relationship with a woman, she replied, "I thought you didn't want to talk about it."

It would be easy to assume that this was purely projection on the part of the patient. She was the one who didn't want to talk about it. I was ready if only she had brought it up. After all, a number of my patients are aware of my sexual orientation and in my personal life I do not keep it a secret. When I gave further thought to this, however, I realized she was right. I hadn't wanted to talk about it. Most of the patients who know that I am a lesbian, are gay or lesbian themselves. If they are heterosexual then they knew of my sexual orientation when they entered treatment and were accepting of it. This is quite different than my bringing the subject to their attention well into our work together.

What would have happened if I had wanted to talk about it or if the patient felt she could raise the issue even if I didn't seem to want to talk about it? Did we miss out on an opportunity to deepen the work? It is a difficult call, whether to introduce these issues into the treatment, or wait for them to come up. However, in this case, my own discomfort was communicated to the patient without my realizing it. Once this information became known, our work shifted significantly. Jamie, who was adopted at birth by a distant and reserved mother, began to talk about her belief that I love the child I gave birth to more than the one that is not biologically my own. This moved to an exploration of what it means to be a mother or to be mothering. What kind of mother could she be, having never felt mothered herself? What kind of mother might I be? What is it like to be a lesbian mother? She spoke of the courage and fear she imagined was involved in my decision to create a family unlike the one I was raised in. She considered the possibility that she too may be able to take the risk of creating something other than what she came from.

WORK WITH LESBIAN PATIENTS

Many of the lesbian patients I was working with had a similar reaction to Jamie's when they learned of my pregnancy. They described my decision to become pregnant as "brave" or "courageous." These patients all knew of my sexual orientation and as a result I was not concerned about the consequences of their finding out that I am a lesbian. This freed me up considerably, allowing me to be more emotionally available and involved in the work. I felt similarly with the heterosexual patients who already knew of my sexual orientation.

Many of the issues that arose with lesbian patients were similar to those that might arise between any pregnant therapist and patient. Depending upon the patient's character, issues such as envy, competition, and abandonment were frequent aspects of the work during this time. For those patients who had felt comforted in the thought that I understood them simply because I too am a lesbian, my pregnancy forced them to recognize our differences. This was especially true for patients who did not want children of their own.

A frequent theme with lesbian patients was related to their perception of their own comfort with their sexual orientation. Many of these patients, upon learning of my pregnancy, began to wonder what it would be like to have to be more publicly known as lesbians and what it would be like for a child to grow up in a gay parented household. For some of these women, the discomfort and anxiety that this caused them was incongruous with their view of themselves as comfortable and confident in their identity as lesbians. In these instances it was important to assess whether their discomfort was connected to their own self-image or whether it was connected to their fears of how they would be treated by others for being gay (Crespi, 1995).

Anna

Anna was a patient for whom many of these issues arose. She is a 29 year old woman who had been in therapy with me for one year prior to learning of my pregnancy. She was extremely successful in her career but had found it difficult to form a satisfying relationship with a partner.

Anna is the younger of two children in a working class Italian family. She describes her childhood home as feeling separate from the rest of the world. At times this separateness felt safe and cocoon like but as she grew older it felt stagnant and deadening. Anna often had the feeling that she was the only one in her family who was really living in the world. Her parents placed great emphasis on their children's academic performances and the development of career goals but they were not particularly concerned with their social lives. They had few relationships with others and seemed to feel social needs and skills were unimportant in life. Anna was a more social and gregarious individual than anyone else in her family. She felt like she was her family's link to life outside her parent's home.

In treatment Anna quickly developed a positive transference and saw me as a connection to a more related world. She thought of therapy as an opportunity for growth and change. This was in sharp contrast to her feelings about her parent's home as a place where "time stood still and nothing could ever grow." Early in treatment Anna often seemed removed and disconnected from what she was talking about during our sessions. It was particularly when feelings of need, anger and isolation would arise that it felt like Anna was floating away. Much of our work has been about helping her to bring her dissociated feelings into awareness.

When Anna learned of my pregnancy she reacted with excitement. She considered it confirmation that I have a life beyond my office and that I am connected to others. Her negative feelings were tied to my leave and the impending separation rather than to the pregnancy itself. I remember feeling pleased that Anna was having such a positive reaction to my pregnancy. It was a relief to have a patient for whom my pregnancy represented hope and a sense of possibility.

Knowing that I am a lesbian, Anna was curious about my decision to become pregnant. She wondered how long I'd thought about it and what went into the planning of my pregnancy. Anna realized that many of the women she'd been involved with had wanted to have a child someday but she had never even considered this as an option for herself. Perplexed by this realization, Anna and I began to explore her dissociated feelings about having a child.

When Anna thought about what it would be like not only to be a mother, but a lesbian mother she felt confused and uneasy. She did not like the idea that if she had a child she would have to be more publicly disclosing about her sexual orientation. She imagined herself dealing with a babysitter, a soccer coach, or the PTA and all of them knowing that she is a lesbian. She felt overwhelmed at the thought of this type of exposure. As Anna spoke it was apparent that she felt none of the things that could be overwhelming for her as a lesbian parent were difficult for me. In Anna's view, I could handle anything. She took comfort in this thought and seemed to feel it was because she had a therapist who was unfazed by all of the challenges that lesbian motherhood presented that she would someday be able to handle being a lesbian mother herself.

I believe two aspects of the transference-countertransference relationship were of particular significance in my work with Anna during this time. One was Anna's need to idealize me. I believe my feelings of vulnerability about being a lesbian mother made it difficult for me to address Anna's idealizing transference to me as someone who could handle anything because, at the time, I wanted to believe that it was true. During my pregnancy I did not want to focus on my fears and anxieties about the medical aspects of the pregnancy, or my fears and anxieties about being a lesbian parent. My need to avoid these areas, which in reality were of great concern to me, made it impossible for me to explore Anna's idealization of me as someone who was entering this new role in a confident and fearless fashion.

The other aspect of the transference-countertransference relationship that grew out of our work during this time was the development of Anna's sense of hope about her own life. After I returned from maternity leave we began a deeper exploration of the transference and her thoughts about my life as a lesbian mother. My ability to have a child and to form a lesbian parented family, in spite of the difficulties and challenges it would present, made Anna look at her own way of living day to day life in a new light, that is, with greater curiosity and, an increased sense of possibility. Sandra Buechler (1995) in her article on hope in psychoanalysis writes,

> I don't believe it is, specifically, the analyst's hope that engenders hope in the patient, but the analyst's whole relationship to life. The patient observes the analyst's struggle to make sense of things, keep going in the face of seemingly insurmountable obstacles, retain humor and courage in situations that seem to inspire neither . . . While in part this attitude may provide a model, and it may be contagious, I think that what mainly creates hope is the patient's experience of finding a way to relate to such a person. (p. 72)

As Anna and I continue our work, it becomes clear that relating to me as someone who has not shied away from the life I want to live, in spite of the challenges it presents, has been a new relational experience for her. Anna's experience of me as someone who can feel vulnerable and overwhelmed by the challenges of my life, but still find pleasure in it, is in sharp contrast to how she sees her family members and, it opens up new possibilities for how she may choose to live her own life.

CONCLUSION

My pregnancy, and the issues of sexual orientation that were linked to it, created an opportunity for my patients and I to explore the meaning of our interactions in ways we never had in the past. With Sarah, Jamie and Anna, as well as other patients, the work deepened, as they were able to talk about their experience of our relationship in a new way. It would not have been possible for me to understand and recognize my patient's feelings about my sexual orientation if I did not allow myself to be aware of and utilize my own countertransferential feelings in this regard (Racker, 1972). It became clear in the work that the formation of close and meaningful relationships was more possible with an exploration and recognition of our differences and similarities rather than a denial of them.

It is my belief that the sexual orientation of the therapist, whether it is disclosed to the patient or not, has a significant impact on the transference-countertransference relationship. My pregnancy forced me to recognize how my countertransferential feelings about my sexual orientation affect my work. My feelings of exposure and of anxiety, hiding, and emotional honesty were all connected with my sexual orientation and how it may have negatively changed my patient's views of me. This left me feeling extremely vulnerable. The degree of vulnerability I experienced was varied, depending upon the patient's familial history and dynamics and on my own relational experience with the patient.

I believe more work needs to be done on homosexuality and countertransference. There must be more room in the profession, in training institutes, supervision settings and in conferences for an exploration of how the gay and lesbian therapist's countertransferential feelings impact the work. Living with the cultural reality that homosexuality is less valued in our society than heterosexuality affects transference and countertransference feelings in the treatment room.

It is only by creating an environment in which gay or lesbian therapists will become more comfortable with their countertransference feelings and with the possibility of their sexual orientation becoming known that they will be able to take more risks with their patients. It is now clear to me that when I am more open and risk taking with my patients, they are more open and risk taking with me. While this may cause me considerable feelings of vulnerability and anxiety, as Stephen Mitchell (1997) states,

> The most interesting and productive moments and periods of analytic work are often precisely those spent outside that familiar, reassuring professional self-times when confusion, dread, excitement, exasperation, longing or passion is the dominant affect. (p. 193)

While it has often been difficult for me to be vulnerable and exposed to my patients, it has been allowing myself to be vulnerable with them in the ways described in this paper that has provided an opportunity for some of our deepest and most intimate work.

BIBLIOGRAPHY

Aron, L. (1996). *A Meeting of Minds*. Hillsdale: NJ: The Analytic Press.

Benedek, E. (1973). The fourth world of the pregnant therapist. *Journal of the American Medical Women's Association, 28*, pp. 365-368

Blechner, M. (1993). Homophobia in Psychoanalytic Writing and Practice. *Psychoanalytic Dialogues* 3:627-37

Buechler, S. (1995). Hope as Inspiration in Psychoanalysis. *Psychoanalytic Dialogues*, 5:63-74

Crespi, L., (1995). Some Thoughts on the Role of Mourning in the Development of a Positive Lesbian Identity. In: *Disorienting Sexuality*, ed. Domenici & Lesser. New York: Routledge, pp. 19-32.

Drescher, J. (1995), Anti-homosexual bias in training. In: Disorienting Sexualities, (ed). Domenici and Lesser. New York: Routledge, pp. 227-241.

Fenster, S., Phillips, S., & Rapoport, E. (1986). *The Therapist's Pregnancy*. New Jersey: Analytic Press.

Frank, K.A. (1997). The Role of the Therapist's Inadvertant Self-Revelations. *Psychoanalytic Dialogues*, 7:281-314

Frommer, M.S. (1995). Countertransference Obscurity. In: *Disorienting Sexuality*, ed. Domenici & Lesser. New York: Routledge, pp. 65-82

Imber, R. (1990). The Avoidance of Countertransference Awareness in a Pregnant Therapist. *Contemporary Psychoanalysis*. 26: 223-236

Magee, M. and Miller, D. (1995). Psychoanalysis and Women's Experiences of "Coming Out." In: *Disorienting Sexuality*, ed. Domenici & Lesser. New York: Routledge, pp. 97-114.

Maroda, K.,(1991). *The Power of Countertransference*. Chichester, UK: Wiley.

Maroda, K. (1999). *Seduction, Surrender and Transformation*. Hillsdale, NJ: The Analytic Press.

Mitchell, S. (1988). *Relational Concepts in Psychoanalysis*. Cambridge, MA: Harvard University Press.

Pines, D. (1972). Pregnancy and Motherhood: Interaction between fantasy and reality. *British Journal of Medical Psychology 45*, pp. 333-343.

Racker, H. (1972). The Meanings and Uses of Countertransference. *Psychoanalytic Quarterly, 41*:487-506.

Renik, O. (1993). Analytic Interaction: conceptualizing technique in light of the therapist's irreducible subjectivity. Psychoanalytic Quarterly, *62*:553-571.

Schwartz, D. (1993). Heterophilia–The Love that Dare Not Speak its Aim. *Psychoanalytic Dialogues, 3*:643-44.

It's a Radical Thing:
A Conversation with April Martin, PhD

Debra Weinstein

SUMMARY. An interview with April Martin, PhD, who has been called "the Dr. Spock of gay parenting" (Raskin, 1993). *[Article copies available for a fee from The Haworth Document Delivery Service: 1-800-342-9678. E-mail address: <getinfo@haworthpressinc.com> Website: <http://Haworth Press.com> © 2001 by The Haworth Press, Inc. All rights reserved.]*

KEYWORDS. Gay, lesbian, parent, transexual, gay rights, psychotherapy, family, birth mother, adoption, transracial, gayby boom

April Martin has been called "the Dr. Spock of gay parenting" (Raskin, 1993). The author of *The Gay and Lesbian Parenting Handbook: Creating and Raising Our Families* (HarperCollins, 1993), she has lectured widely, advocating on behalf of gay families. A psychologist in private practice in New York City, Martin is a member of the supervisory faculty of New York University's Postdoctoral Program in Psychotherapy and Psychoanalysis. Currently she serves on the board of the Family Pride Coalition and is working on their Families and Faith campaign.

We meet on a Sunday afternoon in winter for this interview. Martin's office, in New York City's "fashionably gay" Chelsea section, is comfortably cluttered. Her feet rest on a brown leather animal-faced ottoman, a gift from a former patient.

Debra Weinstein serves as an editor and writer in the School of Education at New York University.

Address correspondence to: Debra Weinstein, New York University, 82 Washington Square East, New York, NY 10003 (E-mail: dbwl@nyu.edu).

[Haworth co-indexing entry note]: "It's a Radical Thing: A Conversation with April Martin, PhD." Weinstein, Debra. Co-published simultaneously in *Journal of Gay & Lesbian Psychotherapy* (The Haworth Medical Press, an imprint of The Haworth Press, Inc.) Vol. 4, No. 3/4, 2001, pp. 63-73; and: *Gay and Lesbian Parenting* (ed: Deborah F. Glazer, and Jack Drescher) The Haworth Medical Press, an imprint of The Haworth Press, Inc., 2001, pp. 63-73. Single or multiple copies of this article are available from The Haworth Document Delivery Service [1-800-342-9678, 9:00 a.m. - 5:00 p.m. (EST). E-mail address: getinfo@haworthpressinc.com].

63

Debra Weinstein: How does having a family with children affect the gay and lesbian identity?

April Martin: I am certainly old enough to remember when there were gays and when there were breeders. We've come a long way since then. The old concept of family left gay people out in the cold. We were presumed not to live in anything that could be called a family. I think this is probably the most dramatic shift: Family issues as of 1999 are spearheading the gay, lesbian, bisexual and transgender civil rights movement along with a widespread community understanding that we live in families. And I would say that shift came hugely as a result of the "gayby" boom. As people began to live in families with children, I think even the broader concept of living in a family without children started to become part of our community identity.

DW: Does this create a generation gap within the gay community?

AM: I think that it is a very different experience coming of age in the 50s or in the early 60s. There are still lots of people in that age group for whom parenting was unthinkable and who arranged their lives and their psychologies in such a way that relating to children through parenting is still unthinkable, if not weird. On the whole, I think there has been a dramatic shift in our community: Young people don't even question that they can become parents, they presume that they can. I don't mean everybody in every rural county, everywhere around the country, but I think in huge numbers young people just presume that some day–if they want to–they can become a parent.

DW: Why do you think that is? What's different?

AM: Visibility. That it's been done. That it's being done. That it shows. That its been talked about. That they can see it being done. That there are resources.

DW: Certainly access to fertility treatment is helpful.

AM: Everything is a result of visibility. The fertility technology has always been there, but it hasn't always been available to single woman until there was the kind of visibility and acceptance of lesbian parent-hood which made doctors and clinics feel okay about it. The same with adoption resources. The more visible we are, the more adoption profes-sionals get to know us as good parents, the broader number of agencies open up to us.

DW: How does being a parent affect the intra-psychic world of the gay person?

AM: It absolutely changes people. Becoming a parent smacks you up against every conflict and unresolved primitive place in you connected to your relationship to your parents. It provides you with a huge challenge to either repeat the damage or overcome it. It's the impetus to grow in a dramatic way. I can't think of anything else that pushes an individual's psychological issues in so profound a way.

DW: You wrote that some suggest that lesbians have children to prove their femininity; men their masculinity. How does having children affect one's sense of internalized homophobia?

AM: I am not sure that there is a generalization you can make about that. I think that some people find it an avenue to more social acceptance, but for other people it forces you to "come out" in ways that are more difficult and challenging. I don't know that those people would say that its an avenue to social acceptance. I think they would say that it is a hard road requiring that you come out all the time and then face opposition.

DW: What about the issue of femininity? How does having a child affect that?

AM: I don't want to fall into the trap of saying that it makes a woman more feminine to be fulfilling the feminine role. But for a lesbian to become a parent adds wonderful richness and depth to the range of gender expression that's possible for her. Not that she becomes more like a heterosexual woman–but lesbian parenting is a radical thing.

DW: How is it a radical thing?

AM: In the mom-and-dad family there is a tremendous emphasis placed on the role of the man and the role of the woman. Theories have been developed for decades about how that is exactly what we need for the development of the child. And these theories have been elaborated in book upon book: Why you need the man's strength and the woman's softness . . . the rivalry with the father, the longing for the mother. All of it has been based on the premise that parenting requires two genders. And now we know that mixed-gender parented families were the only families that the researchers were observing. That they were drawing a lot of conclusions without seeing the full picture.

Lesbian parented families provide a radical perspective on accepted developmental theories. All of our research shows that the children raised in lesbian households are developing indistinguishably from children raised by mixed-gender parents. The gender role expression of the parents doesn't adversely affect the child. It works whether you've got two butch moms, two fem moms, or any variety of gender expression in each of the women. It's radical.

DW: Are there differences between families formed by lesbians and gay men?

AM: Yes, most of the families formed by gay men are formed by adoption.

DW: Do you see the manner in which people have children, whether they give birth or adopt, as having an emotional affect on the individual?

AM: There are a whole range of issues that come with adoption that don't come with biological parenthood. There is the issue of the adopted child's experience of separation from a birth mother. That's a powerful experience with huge ramifications especially if there were many foster homes or long periods of institutional care before the adoption. In families formed by adoption, we have a huge number of transracial issues in our community. But I see surprisingly few differences otherwise. Obviously, you don't have a nursing situation in families formed by adoption, and you might or might not have a nursing situation when somebody gives birth to a child. Gay men who parent by surrogacy aren't nursing their children and some lesbians don't nurse their children anyway.

DW: Nursing changes things?

AM: I don't know that it changes that much. It is a wonderful experience for the nursing couple, but in terms of the family dynamics, does it actually change much? I don't think so. I have seen families where children get very intensely bonded with one parent and go through that phase where they are rejecting of the other parent. I have seen that happen in families where kids have been adopted or been given birth to. I have even seen a child get more intensely bonded to a non-biological mother, when the biological mother had nursed him. So I am not sure that the nursing relationship has all that powerful a meaning. Again, perhaps contrary to lots of our sacred cows of child development.

DW: To be the "other woman" when another mother is nursing is a powerful experience.

AM: To be the "rejected parent" is a horrendous experience and much harder in our families. In mixed-gender parented families, most often it is the dad who is the rejected parent, and there is a cultural support of that. We say "Oh, he wants his mommy." It is understood that the father's role is still important and upheld, and its just natural that a child would prefer a mother's care. In our families there is no institutionalization of that experience. We have no way of saying, "Of course that makes sense, she wants you and not me." It hurts. It is much tougher in our families especially when the rejected mom may be the non-legal parent, the non-biological parent who may have no support from her family for this being her child.

DW: Do lesbian patients ever bring up competitive mothering as an issue in their treatment?

AM: I think all parents compete for the smiles of their children. I think nature planned it that way so that children get as much attention as possible. I see that in every family. I think that's universal.

DW: In families where couples have two children, each conceiving one, do partners ever feel "your kid and my kid?"

AM: Ideally, on any real heart level there should be no sense of "your kid and my kid." There was a family in my practice who were in serious trouble and when they split up, they did it along the lines of "your kid and my kid." And that unfortunately is happening more often in our community. That's a big crisis that we now have to deal with.

DW: There is currently a lot of literature, books, anthologies, e.g., about lesbians raising boys. Do you find lesbians to be a little anxious about raising boys?

AM: Our culture is very concerned about its men. The complaint from the radical right is they don't want two women raising a male child because he won't grow up manly enough. They don't want two men raising a male child because he won't grow up manly enough either. The assumption is that you need a heterosexual man in order to create the right kind of man. Our culture has a certain anxiety about producing those sorts of men.

I think how parents feel about having a son has to do with their own gender stereotyped interests. I had some concerns when I knew I was having a son because I didn't really share those interests. I am not the mom who is going to sit and watch a football game. On the other hand, my partner is. She's thrilled to watch a football game with my son. You hope your kids share your interests in some way. When we chose to have children back in 1980, we were still coming out of the radical feminist 70s with its intense pressure. There was still the stuff about "boys can't come into woman's space, and lesbians should have only girls." We felt some of that. I don't see it now. I see parents thrilled to have either.

But I think that everybody has associations to what it means to be male and female. It think if you polled a lot of straight couples you'd find that they have strong feelings too.

Why is it, though, that of all the concerns people may have about lesbians raising kids, one of most solemn is whether boys will be okay without a male parent?

DW: Dorothy Dinnerstein seemed to think that the devaluation of women would never change as long as boys were raised in heterosexist households. Do you think that the children raised in gay-parented households will change the social order?

AM: I see a remarkable group of kids coming of age who have a sensitivity to diversity and social justice issues. As a group they seem to be very evolved.

DW: Are parenting issues different for gay men and lesbians?

AM: Yes, men take a lot more flack. People just presume that they don't know what is good for a child. The men that I speak to tell me about being intruded on all the time. Walking down the street some woman is bound to stop them and say, "Button up your child's sweater

or don't let him slump like that," presuming that they have no competence as parents. Two men with a small child arouse suspicion more
than two women with a small child. I have friends who got pulled over
by the police because they were two men driving in a car with a little
girl in the back seat. Somebody was sure that they had kidnapped her.

DW: Do your patients mourn the inability to conceive with their partners?

AM: I think that people are sad not to be able to create a child that is a
genetic combination of themselves and their partner, but I don't see
anybody upset that they can't do it by having sex. I think that is a
non-issue. Sex is just as good if it doesn't make a baby. A baby is just
as good if it didn't happen when you had sex.

DW: Recently I read that every child is born out of her parent's desire–

AM: Desire to parent–not born out of the desire for sex. There's
nothing about one's lust that prepares one for parenthood. I think that
is a terribly romantic notion. The idea that there is something better
about creating a child through your sexual passion seems pretty use-
less to me.

DW: Conception isn't so important?

AM: It sure isn't. It has been elevated to a cultural notion that needs to
be debunked.

DW: How do your patients work though the inability to have children
with their partners?

AM: There are some lesbian couples that use one woman's egg and
implant in the other, so the other one can give birth to her partner's
baby. Using a brother's sperm does give you a genetic combination,
but it often turns out to be messy. (People don't do that so often.) I've
seen interracial couples where a white partner will use a black donor
and vice versa. I think the range of biological possibilities makes it so
that you have to raise the question: How important is biology? Clearly
in our families biology can't be as important as in the families that
heterosexuals create. We don't have the same options. But I think we

find that on an emotional/psychological level, biology turns out to be not as important. Ultimately, we come up with the answer that it means very little in the bigger picture of what it takes to raise a child 24 hours a day/7 days a week for 20 years.

DW: You are a pioneer in the gay parenting movement. Where is the movement going and where do you think it has been?

AM: Where we came from: we are standing on the shoulders of the early homophile movement, the women's movement, the movement for black civil rights. Without those giants, the "gayby" boom generation would not exist.

Where we're going: I think the issue of transgender parenting is a quite profound. The movement is at least paying lip service now to inclusiveness: Gays, lesbians, bisexuals and transgenders, that's our mantra now. I think we need a lot more visibility for transgender issues. I think we need to get away from identity politics: I am a lesbian, she is a transgendered person. I think we need to stop focusing on identity politics and stop making the argument that "we deserve our civil rights because we can't help who we are; we can't change who we are; it has a genetic basis. I think that's the wrong argument. I think that we are evolving toward an argument of behavior politics: We deserve our civil rights because there is no dress code for civil rights. Who I love, how I love, what I wear, what occupation I choose, should not impact on my civil rights.

I think that in many ways the transgendered community is contributing a tremendous piece of what will be a tidal wave shift in that direction. Because at the bottom of homophobia is gender politics. The intolerance that our culture has had toward a diversity of gender role expression is what we need to change. Ultimately I hope we get to the place where every kid can grow up believing that they can be whoever they want to be gender-wise. They can love whoever they want to love and they can parent if and when they want to parent.

Visibility is the issue. The studies show that the more people see us the more their fear about us and their stereotyping is reduced.

DW: What are some of special problems that transgendered people have raising children?

AM: I think that one of the huge problems for kids whose parents have changed their assigned gender is that there is not enough community for them yet or enough visibility. It means that every place they go they are having to make a lot of explanations; they have to come out without support. There are courageous pioneers doing this all over the country, but they need to have more organization behind them. The children of people who have changed their assigned gender are in the position that kids with gay parents were in 20 years ago.

DW: I noticed you have pictures of your children in your office. Can you talk a little about your work as an analyst and what it might mean to have their pictures here?

AM: My work is analytically informed. I do very, very in-depth work with many people. How many times a week depends more on their finances and their time. I don't subscribe to the idea of the analyst as a blank slate. I think that to imagine you are a blank slate is to lie to yourself. There are things that will always be known about you. If you withhold everything, the thing that's known about you is that you are withholding. I think you might as well say who you are and deal with the things people project onto that or interpret that. The important meaning of the analyst as blank slate is more that the analyst does not bring her need system into the relationship. That the relationship be focused on the needs of the patient and the analyst merely bring her needs to get paid, not her need for emotional nourishment in any way.

I made the decision to put the pictures of my kids in this room, and certainly there are lots of things in this room that show who I am. Aside from my degrees, there are my books. Anybody looking at my books knows who I am. Anyone looking at my messy desk knows who I am. The AIDS quilt on my wall. So, I am not trying to hide who I am. But I made the decision to put my kids' pictures here because–I did this when they were very young–I felt that the visibility issue was tremendously important. Eighty percent of my practice is gay and lesbian. I still see people who have never seen or don't know of a long-term happy gay relationship. I feel like they need to know; they need to see us. They need to see that we live in families. It's terribly sad to see a young person who thinks that gay relationships don't last more than six months because they are only travelling in a peer group where that's true. They haven't grown up with a visible long-term gay couple or older role models. They need to know that it is possible in the world.

DW: I think it is a very strong statement: out, lesbian, mother. That's what you're saying, I think.

AM: Yes, and it doesn't stop transference. The people who are going to idealize you for that are going to idealize you. The people who are going to find in you all the things they most fear or had difficulty with in their parents–that you're untrustworthy, that you're inattentive–they're going to find those things.

DW: Well, they're not going to have a fantasy that they're your only child.

AM: That's true, but that doesn't stop them from having a fantasy that they're my most important relationship or that they're my least important relationship.

DW: In reference to your book, where you use your own journey to parenthood as illustration and example–how does having personal information out in the world affect the treatment?

AM: I think that people have to do as therapists what they're comfortable with. I know therapists who are most comfortable not having to deal with people's projections that really involve real information about their lives. I've had patients who have used the information that they know about me to comment on my cancelling an appointment. That puts the therapist in a very vulnerable position. If somebody wants to attack me and has real pieces of data, it becomes my job to keep the distance and recognize that what a patient is doing with the information is about him and not about me. I feel comfortable to do that. I understand that some therapists don't feel comfortable to do that. I prefer that people have that information about me probably because I spent too much of life lying and hiding who I was. I don't want to do that anymore.

    Among the patients that I see there are some who want to know more about you and some that never want you to say anything about yourself. I will accommodate to either and will consider that an important question to address: why do they want to know and why do they not want to know? Somebody who really wants to have a sense of a therapist as a non-person is not going to come to me. I don't think every therapist can treat every patient.

DW: What can therapy do for gay people?

AM: The kind of work that needs to be done with gays and lesbians is exactly the work you do with an abused child. However, the issue for gay people is cultural abuse.

Those of us who grew up lesbian, gay, bisexual or transgendered, have been chronically, subtly, pervasively demeaned, insulted, threatened, vilified, and grossly neglected by our cultures. If this behavior were perpetrated on us by another person we would call it abuse. We respond to it the same way as we respond to personal abuse: We believe we deserve it and we stay attached to the society that perpetrates it, sometimes even echoing and advocating homophobic sentiments.

When we were abused as children–physically, sexually, emotionally–we had little choice but to internalize the violence and form some kind of internal connection to the abusive party. The task of therapy is to clearly identify this interaction between person and culture as abuser. The aim is to liberate the self from bondage with a demeaning and threatening culture. As we help free each person to value themselves for their intrinsic worth, they can let go of the need for approval from a destructive culture. This will open the door to making attachments to people who are loving and supportive.

Legal Issues Affecting Alternative Families:
A Therapist's Primer

Carol Buell, Esq.

SUMMARY. When heterosexuals fall in love, get married and have children, the last thing on their mind is taking legal steps to protect their family. In seeing their lesbian and gay clients, therapists will often notice the same thing. However, at the moment when one's mind is least focused on legal matters, lesbian and gay couples must focus on protecting their relationships through wills, health care proxies, and advanced directives and must focus on protecting their children through second parent adoptions, known donor agreements or other kinds of agreements. This article will outline the kinds of legal issues you must isolate for your clients so that they can legalize their relationships and families. *[Article copies available for a fee from The Haworth Document Delivery Service: 1-800-342-9678. E-mail address: <getinfo@haworthpressinc.com> Website: <http://www.HaworthPress.com> © 2001 by The Haworth Press, Inc. All rights reserved.]*

KEYWORDS. Adoption, second parent adoption, gay, lesbian, family, donor insemination, surrogate mothers, law

There are an estimated 6-10 million lesbian and gay parents in the United States. These gay and lesbian parents are the fathers and mothers of an estimated 14 million children throughout this country. Al-

---

Carol Buell, Esq., is a partner in the law firm of Weiss, Buell, and Bell, New York, NY.

Address correspondence to: Carol Buell, Esq., 350 Fifth Avenue, Suite 2604, New York, NY 10018 (E-mail: cbuell@wbblaw.com).

[Haworth co-indexing entry note]: "Legal Issues Affecting Alternative Families: A Therapist's Primer." Buell, Carol. Co-published simultaneously in *Journal of Gay & Lesbian Psychotherapy* (The Haworth Medical Press, an imprint of The Haworth Press, Inc.) Vol. 4, No. 3/4, 2001, pp. 75-90; and: *Gay and Lesbian Parenting* (ed: Deborah F. Glazer, and Jack Drescher) The Haworth Medical Press, an imprint of The Haworth Press, Inc., 2001, pp. 75-90. Single or multiple copies of this article are available from The Haworth Document Delivery Service [1-800-342-9678, 9:00 a.m. - 5:00 p.m. (EST). E-mail address: getinfo@haworthpressinc.com].

75

though many of these children were born when their parents were in heterosexual relationships, the last decade has seen a sharp rise among lesbians and gays planning and forming families through adoption, foster care, donor insemination, and other reproductive technologies. Some have described the current trend as the lesbian and gay baby boom. As your clients seek help in making decisions about whether to start a family, there are a number of legal issues of which you should be aware. In this article I will provide an overview of the types of legal documents your client should have in order to protect their relationships and their children. These documents include a will, health care proxy or living will, advanced directives, such as Nomination of Guardian or Conservators, powers of attorney and medical authorizations. The remainder of the article deals with legal issues facing your clients should they create their families by means such as alternative insemination, surrogacy or adoption. In addition, this article will discuss legal issues affecting your clients and families when breaking up, such as custody and visitation.

I. PROTECTION OF THE RELATIONSHIP

In every area of the country the laws are clear about who is entitled to your estate upon your death. If you have not executed a Will, the law of the state in which you reside will determine who is entitled to your estate based upon marital status only. Married couples are considered each other's next of kin, whether a Will has been executed or not. If one is not married, then your next of kin is typically your children (if any), your parents, siblings or nieces and nephews, in that order. Lesbian and gay partners are considered legal strangers and will not inherit each other's property unless they have signed Wills.

In addition to Wills, each partner should consider documents which protect the relationship and give control to the partner prior to death but during their incapacity from health or mental reasons. These items, referred to as "advanced directives" enable you to determine who would make financial and medical decisions in the event of incapacity. Documents such as Nominations of Guardian or Conservators, Powers of Attorney, and Living Wills and Health Care Proxies all enable your clients to appoint partners to make these decisions.

II. CREATING OUR FAMILIES

A. Alternative Insemination (AI)

There are three ways AI can be performed. The first way is AIH, i.e., insemination when the recipient's husband is the donor. This technique need not be discussed in the context of lesbian relationships. The second technique is called AIC: insemination by both unrelated donor and husband combined. *To the extent that it involves marital relations, this technique need not be discussed in the context of lesbian relationships. However, your lesbian and gay clients may want to consider paternity issues that arise when two donors combine their sperm.* The third technique is AID: insemination when sperm from a donor, whether known or unknown, is used. *This technique applies to lesbians creating families, and AID is really the only technique relevant to the article.*

How does conception through AI affect the parental rights of lesbian families? Generally, a husband who consents to the AI of his wife using sperm of a third party donor is treated as the father of the child. Moreover, the father will likely incur the obligation to support the child if the marriage dissolves (A.L.R.4th 295, 1991). For same-sex couples, however, because there is no legal right to marry, presumptions of obligation and parenthood do not apply. To gain parental rights the non-biological mother must petition the court for second parent adoption. (See adoption section.) If the bio mother's partner has not petitioned for adoption of the child and the relationship dissolves, in order for the bio mother to claim that her partner has parental responsibilities and obligations, the bio mother must rely upon a co-parenting agreement. Such an agreement outlines the partners' intent to raise the child together as their own. A co-parenting agreement will probably be enforceable against the nonbio/legal mother if the bio mother asserts that her partner has an obligation to support the child. However, there are no reported cases in legal treatises (case law) on this point, probably because most of these types of disputes get settled outside of the courts. In typical co-parenting agreements the attorney/ draftsperson will add clauses which enable the parents to seek non-litigious options to settle their disputes such as mediation or arbitration. In many areas of the country lesbian and gay communities have begun mediation projects to assist lesbian and gay families in these types of disputes. (See custody and visitation section for more information.)

Many of your clients will be struggling with whether to use a known or unknown donor for purposes of AI. Most attorneys would agree that there are some benefits of knowing the identity of the donor but many legal risks. In using a known donor, medical information and history can be useful to address health problems that the child might face. In addition some children may wish to know the identity of the donor. Finally many women may be better able to screen the sperm of a known donor because some sperm banks may be unreliable. These benefits must be weighed against the very real risks that a donor may assert parental rights. When the donor of the semen is known to the recipient, the donor and the recipient usually enter into a contract under which the donor agrees not to assert any parental rights and the recipient agrees not to assert the rights of the child to receive child support. These contracts may also delineate the donor's role in the child's life, i.e., visitation rights. So long as the parties adhere to the contract, there are no problems; however, if there is a violation of the agreement, the parties may find themselves in court. The court is required to examine whether the contract is enforceable and valid, whether the non-biological parent/partner has standing to assert her parenthood, whether the sperm donor has standing to assert paternity, and whether parental status is determined by biology or socialization. There is much debate however, about whether any of these donor agreements will be enforceable in court since any agreement effecting a child may be voidable by the court if the court perceives that it is not in the child's best interest. An agreement between the parties to resolve disputes through mediation and/or arbitration is very important.

Because of the risks in using a known donor many lesbian couples choose to use unknown donors. The National Center for Lesbian Rights recommends these guidelines to lesbians who are planning to have children through artificial insemination: (1) use an anonymous donor, (2) comply with state statute provisions which sever the sperm donor's rights, (3) sign a written agreement with a known sperm donor that he will not have any parental rights or obligations, (4) do not allow a relationship to develop between the known donor and the child, and (5) do not act inconsistently with severance of the sperm donor's parental rights.

If your client is contemplating becoming a known donor it would be advisable to explore all of his motivations. If he truly wants to be a parent in every sense of the word, rather than just a "distant uncle," he may be hurt by this process. On the other hand, many lesbians and gays are interested in breaking out of social constructs and forming different families, children with three or four parents, for example. While it may be possible for some of our clients to accomplish this utopian goal, it is imperative that lesbian and gay practitioners, whether in a legal or therapeutic context, work closely with our clients to help them understand their motivations so that they aren't hurt in the process (or more importantly the children-to-be are not the pawns in a very real legal dispute if the utopian goals fail).

Are there any laws in any state which protect our families? The answer is No. A majority of states have enacted legislation to address AI. The language of the Uniform Parentage Act ("UPA"), adopted by most jurisdictions, addresses "married women" only (Wray, 1997, 127, 137). The UPA, and the statutes enacting its language, fail to clarify the donor's relationship to a child of an unmarried (or lesbian) woman.

B. Surrogacy Issues

When counseling gay men and their partners on how to create their families inevitably the issue of surrogacy will arise. "Surrogate parenting" or "surrogacy" refers to a contract in which the "biological" or surrogate mother agrees, for a fee, to conceive a child through artificial insemination with the sperm of the "biological" father, to bear and deliver the child, then to terminate all parental rights after the child is born (77 A.L.R.4th 70, 1991).

Many gay men have approached friends and family members to discuss the possibility of creating a family by having a woman carry a child on his behalf or his partner's behalf. Many gay men are not aware that surrogacy arrangements are illegal in many states. Several states have enacted statutes that expressly prohibit the enforcement of surrogate parenting agreements, and others have introduced bills to regulate or prohibit them (77 A.L.R.4th 70, 1991). The Uniform Status of Children of Assisted Conception Act of 1988 ("USCACA") provides the basis for most state surrogacy statutes. Marla J. Hollandsworth (1995, 183, 197) divides these surrogacy statutes into three groups:

1. those that completely prohibit surrogacy (and maybe even criminalize surrogacy), despite the USCACA,

2. those that regulate surrogacy arrangements,

- e.g., New Hampshire Surrogacy Statute: enacted in 1990. A surrogacy arrangement is legal only if it is judicially preauthorized. This authorization only comes after all parties complete both medical and non-medical evaluations and attend counseling sessions. Also the contract must conform to certain requirements which annunciate the rights of the parties. The court must also determine whether the agreement is in the best interests of the child. *(See,* also, Ferguson, 1995, 924),

3. those that render surrogacy contracts void and unenforceable, thereby providing no recourse in the courts, but not precluding parties from entering into the arrangements.

- e.g., NY Domestic Relations Law §121: declares that surrogate parenting contracts are contrary to public policy and are void and unenforceable. There will be a civil penalty and forfeiture to the state of any fee received by the surrogate. There is an exception, however, for payments to the surrogate to cover medical costs. 45 NY Jur. 2d Domestic Relations § 347 (1995).
- These statutes provide no legal recourse to gay men considering surrogacy should a "legal nightmare" occur when a surrogate changes her mind (Ferguson, *1995, 903).* If the surrogate changes her mind, and the parties find themselves in litigation for custody, the litigation will be governed by the "best interests of the child" standard. As exemplified by the area of gay and lesbian adoption and custody, this standard is subjective and not always favorable to gay men and lesbians.
- c.f. "Although various court battles over surrogacy arrangements have received widespread media attention, *only one percent* of surrogate mothers change their minds and decide to keep the child" (Ferguson, ibid.).

There is much debate in the lesbian and gay legal community about whether surrogacy arrangements are a valid way of creating our families. Proponents of surrogacy argue it is merely the flip side of lesbians conceiving through AI. In many surrogacy situations no money changes hands. The woman consents to bearing the child because she is a friend, family member or someone who understands that this is the only way the gay man can have a child of his own. On the other hand, one cannot equate a man donating sperm to a woman, with a woman who must carry a child for nine months and create physical risks to herself. What the therapist needs to understand is that surrogacy arrangements can have legal and emotional complications for all parties involved.

C. Adoption

Overview

Many lesbians and gay men are creating their families by means of adoption. There are two types of adoptions that your clients might be discussing with you. One is second parent adoption and the other is agency or private adoption which is the more traditional adoption.

What Is Adoption? While the specific procedures and substantive law of adoption differ state to state, the petition process is generally the same. The person(s) who wants to adopt files a petition in the appropriate court, i.e., Family or Surrogate's Court. The Court then reviews the petition, which usually involves a home investigation study by a "disinterested" party. Other parties are given notice and the right to contest–usually the relatives of the child to be adopted. The state may contest the adoption if it thinks that the person petitioning to adopt is "parentally unfit" (Lambda, p. 1).

Florida is the only state that expressly prohibits lesbians and gay men from adopting children. The statute says that "No person eligible to adopt under the statute may adopt if that person is a homosexual." New Hampshire is cited in the literature as the other state that expressly bans gay men and lesbians from adopting, but this part of the statute was recently repealed (Freiberg, 1999, 1, 11). Courts look to the language of the state's statute on "who may adopt" and interpret the statute as either denying or permitting adoptions by lesbians and gay men.

If the court interprets the statute to allow adoption by a lesbian or gay man, the standard of review is the "best interests of the child." Differences occur in what states/judges consider the best interests of the child; the sexual orientation of the petitioner has been used in some cases to find the adoption *not* in the best interests of the child.

Many of your clients are adopting through traditional means, either through an agency or through a private placement adoption. An agency adoption is the adoption of a foster child who has been in custody and care of an adult for a certain amount of time specified by statute. A private placement adoption is carried out without the direct involvement of the state. It usually takes the form of an adoption through privately run licensed adoption agencies, adoptions of children of family members or friends where the biological parents have either died or consented, or adoptions of foreign orphans brought into the U.S. with permission of the Immigration and Naturalization Service (INS).

Agency Adoptions

Agency Adoption: Most states allow either an unmarried individual or a couple to become foster parents. When the foster child becomes eligible for adoption, the foster parent(s) are generally given preference if he/she/they wish to adopt the foster child. Lesbians and gay men may apply individually (i.e., not as a couple) to become a foster parent, then, when the child is eligible for adoption, the couple may jointly apply to adopt the child.

- All states permit unmarried individuals to become foster parents and to adopt. Many states, either through the courts or the legislature, have ruled that the sexual orientation of the parent should not be considered *unless* it is shown to be harmful to the child, in a way other than societal stigmatization. This finding is up to the judge, and the judge's opinions may affect what s/he views as in the best interests of the child. The judge on the case may greatly affect whether the adoption is granted.
- In Florida, gay men and lesbians can be foster parents because the statute only prohibits "homosexuals" from *adopting*. The Ohio Supreme Court held that a gay man could adopt a child who he had counseled as a psychologist. The Ohio court determined that adoption cases should be decided on a case by case basis, and that gay men and lesbians should not be prohibited from adopting as a matter of law. (The Adoption had been challenged by the Department of Human Services.) *In Re Charles B.*, 552 N.E.2d 884 (Ohio 1990). Also, a New Jersey court allowed two men to adopt a baby boy (Markey, 1998, 721).

Private Placement

Private placement adoptions do not involve the same risks as agency adoptions where the state has the primary goal of reuniting the children with their parents; however, the legal hurdles for approval by the state are largely the same. (Lambda Overview, pg. 5)

- Even privately arranged adoptions must be approved by the court and generally require a home study. The standard is the same as all other adoptions: the best interests of the child.

a. *Private Agency*: The private agency arranging the adoption must do an in-depth investigation of the fitness of the applicants. Because some private adoption agencies are more gay and lesbian friendly in their fitness investigations, you should counsel your clients to contact the local gay and lesbian organizations and adoption information services.

- There are no known cases of a gay or lesbian couple challenging the decision of a private adoption agency. (Private agencies are "quasi-governmental entities" so they *may be* liable if they discriminate based on sexual orientation; however, it is easy for the private agency to hide the discrimination by simply providing grounds other than sexual orientation for refusing to accept gays and lesbians as clients, or for determining that the adoption is not in the best interests of the child.)

b. *Interfamilial Adoption*: Must be approved by the court, and can be contested by the state child welfare agency. The courts have historically granted gay men and lesbians the adoption of a child of a family member. While such adoptions may be denied, an interfamilial adoption, especially of an orphaned child, heightens the court's tolerance of the petitioner's sexuality.

Adoption of Foreign, Orphaned Children

A prospective adoptive parent must apply to the Immigration and Naturalization Service (INS) for advance processing of the orphan petition. When the orphan visa petition is granted, it permits the prospective adoptive parents to bring the child into the U.S. Screening for parental fitness may or may not occur in the child's home country. The Administrative Appeals Unit of INS has declared that any prospective adoptive parent's personal relationships with other adults (i.e., his/her sexual orientation) cannot serve as a basis for a denial of an orphan visa petition.

In recent years many countries have closed the door on adoptions by "known homosexuals." Many agencies specializing in international adoptions must make express statements to the country's representatives that a prospective adoptive parent is not gay or lesbian. Your clients should know that their application to the child's home country may have to be as a single parent. Once again you should counsel your clients to contact a local lesbian and gay organization for information.

Second Parent Adoption

A second parent adoption is achieved through a petition by a lesbian or gay (non-legal/biological) parent to legally adopt the biological/legal child/children of his/her partner, much like step-parent situation in the family of a heterosexual couple. Your client may or may not be able to adopt his or her partner's child depending upon in which state your client resides. In some states it has been clearly determined by the highest court in the state.

In many other states the right to have a second parent adoption has not been determined by the highest court in that state. However, intermediate court decisions have permitted second parent adoptions. If your clients live in New Jersey, Illinois, or Washington DC they may be able to successfully second parent adopt in their area, but should consult a local attorney. Finally lower courts in many other states, have approved second parent adoptions on a case by case basis. But since no intermediate court has approved the adoption in an appeal situation, there is no precedential value to all of those cases. Again clients must seek local legal counsel familiar with second parent adoptions. Some states have entirely disapproved adoptions by gay men and lesbians (Florida, Alabama and Wisconsin). Second parent adoptions are, as are all adoptions by gay men and lesbians, expressly prohibited by Florida statutes. In the past, lesbians and gay men were denied petitions to adopt their partner's children based on the strict reading of adoption statutes which use words such as "spouse" and "stepparent." Because the civil marriage of same-sex couples was not, and is still not, recognized by any of the states, a strict reading of an adoption statute does not allow gays and lesbians to adopt, as they cannot legally become a "spouse" or "stepparent." As no state permits gay and lesbian couples to marry, the issue in second-parent adoptions has become whether the existing legal/biological parent loses legal/parental rights when the adoption of the child by their partner is approved. Some courts have denied petitioners' adoption requests because the biological/legal parent did not want to terminate his/her legal rights, which is a prerequisite to adoption under the statute (Lambda Adoption Overview pg 2).

Highest State Court Decisions Permitting Second Parent Adoptions: The highest state courts in New York, Vermont and Massachusetts have permitted lesbians and gay men to adopt the children of their partners without extinguishing the legal rights of the partner/legal parent. The law in these 3 states now resembles the law for stepparent adoptions of a spouse's child/children. (While these adoptions by gays and lesbians are permitted, they can still be contested by third parties as well as the state child welfare agency) (Lambda Adoption Overview, ibid.).

- Vermont: *In re Adoption of B.L.V.B.*, 628 A.2d 1271 (Vt. 1993).
- Massachusetts: *Adoption of Tammy*, 619 N.E.2d 315 (Mass. 1993).
- New York: *In re Jacob, In re Dana* 660 N.E. 2d391 (N.Y. 1995)

Intermediate Court Decisions Permitting Second Parent Adoptions: Appellate Courts in New Jersey, Illinois and Washington, D.C. have permitted Second Parent adoptions by gay and lesbian partners. These adoptions are not opposed, and thus, have not been appealed, giving them precedential value for lower courts in these states (Lambda Adoption Overview, ibid.). In other words your client may able to petition in some counties in this state, but not all.

Lower Courts Approving Second Parent Adoptions: Alabama, Alaska (Juneau), California (many counties), Colorado, Indiana, Iowa, Maryland, Michigan (selected counties), Minnesota (Aitkin and Hennepin Counties), Nevada, New Mexico, Ohio (several counties), Oregon (Multnomah County), Pennsylvania (York), Rhode Island, Texas (San Antonio), and Washington (King County). These court rulings do not hold precedential value, and those gay men and lesbians considering second parent adoption should contact the local bar or lesbian and gay parenting organization in their state (Lambda Adoption Overview, pg. 3, *especially footnote 4.*).

States Disapproving Second Parent Adoption: Florida, Alabama and Wisconsin disapprove of adoption by gay men and lesbians. Second parent adoptions, as all adoptions by gay men and lesbians, are expressly prohibited by Florida Statute (see background section above). Likewise, in Act 98-439, HJR 35, the Alabama legislature passed a joint resolution stating "that we hereby express our intent to prohibit child adoption by homosexual couples." Wisconsin's Supreme Court strictly interpreted the language of its statute to hold that, even if the adoption was in the best interests of the child, the legal/biological mother had to extinguish all parental rights for her partner to adopt her child because the couple could (can) not get married. In *Re Interest of Angel Lace M.*, 516 N.W.2d 678 (Wis. 1994). A Colorado appellate court held that an unmarried lesbian mother could not consent to adoption of her natural child by her partner without terminating her legal/parental rights. *Matter of Adoption of T.K.J.*, 931 P.2d. 488 (Co. App. 1996). A Connecticut court held that a lesbian could adopt her partner's child without forcing the biological mother to extinguish her legal/parental rights *only if* the couple applied for, and received, a waiver of certain requirements of the statute from the "adoption review board." *In re Adoption of Baby Z*, 699 A.2d 1065 (1996).

Joint Custody Granted to Lesbian Couple Before the Child is Born: A lesbian couple in California were recently granted joint custody of their son before he was born (by an openly gay judge of the Superior Court). One of the women gave birth to the child after undergoing an expensive in vitro fertilization to become pregnant. The egg, which was fertilized by an unknown donor and implanted into one of the women came from her partner. The couple's attorney distinguished their legal action from that of an adoption because both women are the child's parents from conception (Smith, 1, 11).

A Personal Perspective: Deborah Lashman, the non-biological parent in the second parent adoption that rose to the Supreme Court of Vermont (Lashman, 1995, 227), writes a good explanation of "what it was like to go through the legal process [of adoption] as a parent." The article gives a good idea of what it must be like to be a test-case—knowing that the outcome of your case will affect the legal rights of gay and lesbian families in your state. Many of the legal overviews on this issue talk about second-parent adoption as a gay or lesbian person adopting their partner's children. This article is important because it discusses how the petitioning parent is often already the child's parent in every way but legally.

Given the legal impediments and potential costs* of second parent adoptions, many clients may be struggling with their decision about whether to proceed with a second parent adoption. Legal Scholar Karen Markey (1998, 721) outlines some of the potential benefits:

- Serves child by conferring legal responsibility on the parent to support the child.
- The legal parent may make medical decisions for the child.
- The child may inherit from the legal parent, and receive social security benefits.
- Allows child to live with legal parent in the event that the biological parent dies.
- The child may receive health benefits from parent's employer.
- Provides continuity in child's life: gives legal parent standing to petition for custody or visitation in the event that the parents break up.

(*vary from $2,000-$10,000, depending on circumstances)

III. CUSTODY AND VISITATION

Much has been written about gay and lesbian parents seeking custody or visitation of children after the dissolution of a heterosexual relationship in which the parties were legally married. The parties in these "traditional" custody battles resolve custody and visitation issues in the court system of their local communities. The court (judge) has broad discretionary power to grant or deny custody to a parent because such determination is to be based on the best interests of the child. But how are custody and visitation issues resolved in same sex unions? A determination by a judge of what is in the best interest of a child is never made. Custody and visitation settlements are not subject to the review of the courts for gays and lesbians since they cannot be legally married. Nevertheless, gay and lesbian couples dissolve their relationship just as heterosexual couples, but unlike their straight counterparts, the nonlegal parent will not be able to rely on the court system to assist the "family" on custody and visitation issues. The lesbian and gay community is struggling with what to do about the legal parent "pulling rank" and denying visitation to the nonlegal parent. In other instances, nothing prevents the nonlegal parent from leaving the family and refusing to support the child brought into the "intact" lesbian and gay family, even if the decision to raise the child was a mutual one.

In states where second parent adoption is not possible, practitioners should encourage their clients to negotiate and sign co-parenting agreements. (See alternative insemination section for discussion of these agreements.)

The reality is that very few of our clients anticipate the possibility of the dissolution of their relationship when they are planning their families. It is the farthest thing from their minds and they would vehemently state that they would never "pull rank" on their partner. We all know that our clients behave differently when they are breaking up. The challenge for the lesbian and gay community is to deal effectively with the children of these dissolutions and establish social and moral codes for coping with these challenges, while striving to change the laws to protect our families and the children of the families. A coalition of practitioners and lawyers, mediators and parents recently published "standards" for child custody disputes in same sex relationships. Published by Gay and Lesbian Advocates & Defenders in Boston (with the assistance of Lambda Legal Defense & Education Fund, Inc., The National Center for Lesbian Rights, Family Pride Coalition, and the ACLU's Lesbian and Gay Rights Project), the 10 recommendations make very specific suggestions regarding steps the community should follow when dealing with child custody issues. While the document is too extensive to set forth here, it is a good first step in dealing with the very real issues our community is facing.

IV. CONCLUSION

Decisions about whether to become a parent are not easy ones for lesbian and gay clients. There are no unplanned children. All children are intentionally conceived or adopted and it is our job to assist our clients not only with the emotional roller coaster that is the road toward parenthood, but the legal challenges as well. While it is not the job of the therapist to give legal advice, it is important to understand these issues and to discuss them with your clients. For your lesbian and gay clients, unlike straight couples choosing to parent, the emotional issues are only half of the equation. If gay and lesbian parents don't protect their relationships and their children through Wills, second parent adoptions, donor and co-parenting agreements, the courts will not and cannot intervene in the event of death of a loved one or dissolution of a relationship.

REFERENCES

ACLU Fact Sheet: Overview of Lesbian and Gay Parenting, Adoption and Foster Care, <.aclu.org/isses/gay/parent.html>. *See also*, attached, *Overview of State Adoption Laws*, from Lambda Adoption Overview pgs. 8-12 (note: this list is from 1996 and needs to be updated).

Capron, A.M. and M.J. Radin (1990), *Choosing Family Law Over Contract Law as a Paradigm for Surrogate Motherhood*, from Surrogate Motherhood, ed. Larry Gostin, p. 62.

Consent of Natural Parents as Essential to Adoption Where Parents Are Divorced, 47 A.L.R.2d 824 (1956).

Donor Rights in Situations Involving Unmarried Recipients, 26 J. Fam. L. 793 (1988)

Ferguson, Susan A. (1995), *Surrogacy Contracts in the 1990's: The controversy and Debate Continues*, 33 Duq. L.Rev., pp. 903, 904 (explaining gestational surrogacy).

45 NY Jur.2d Domestic Relations § 347 (1995).

Hollandsworth, Marla J. (1995), *Gay Men Creating Families Through Surro-Gay Arrangements: A Paradigm For Reproductive Freedom*, 3 Am. U. J. Gender & L., pp. 183, 197.

Karin T. v. Michael T., 484 NYS2d 780 (1985). *See Rights and Obligations Resulting from Human Artificial Insemination*, 83 A.L.R.4th 295 (1991).

Kerian, Christine L. (1997), *Surrogacy: A Last Resort Alternative For Infertile Women or A Commodification Women's Bodies and Children?*, Wis Women's L.J., pp. 113, 114.

Lambda Legal Defense and Education Fund, *Adoption By Lesbians and Gay Men: An Overview of the Law in the 50 States*, p 1 (hereinafter referred to as "Lambda Adoption Overview.").

Lambda, *Lesbian and Gay Parenting: A Fact Sheet*, <.lambdalegal.org/cgi-bin/pages/documents/record?record=31>.

Lashman, Deborah (1995), *Second Parent Adoption: A Personal Perspective*, 2 Duke J. Gender L. & Poly, pp. 227.

Macklin, Ruth (1990), *Is There Anything Wrong With Surrogate Motherhood?: An Ethical Analysis*, from Surrogate Motherhood, ed. Larry Gostin, p. 142.

Markey, Karen (1998), Note, *An Overview of the Legal Challenges Faced by Gay and Lesbian Parents: How Courts Treat The Growing Number of Gay Families*, 14 N.Y.L. Sch. J. Hum. Rts., pp. 721, 746, 750.

NH ST s 170-B:4; *see also* Freiberg, Peter (April 23, 1999), *Gay Adoption Ban Repealed*, New York Blade News, Vol. 3 No. 17, pgs 1, 11.

Rights and Obligations Resulting from Human Artificial Insemination, 83 A.L.R.4th 295 (1991).

Smith, Rhonda (April 23, 1999), *Lesbians Win Joint Custody*, New York Blade News, Vol. 3 No. 17, pgs. 1, 11.

This Child Does Have Two Mothers . . . And a Sperm Donor With Visitation," 22 N.Y.U. Rev. L. & Soc. Change 1, 27-37 (1996).

Wray, Tsippi (1997), *Lesbian Relationships and Parenthood: Models for Legal Recognition of Nontraditional Families*, 21 Hamline L. Rev., pp. 127, 136. *See Leckie v. Voorhies*, 875 P.2d 521 (Or. Ct. App. 1994).

Families of the Lesbian Baby Boom: Maternal Mental Health and Child Adjustment

Charlotte J. Patterson, PhD

SUMMARY. This article reports a study of maternal mental health, household composition, and children's adjustment among 37 families in which 4- to 9-year-old children had been born to or adopted early in life by lesbian mothers. Results showed that maternal reports of both self-esteem and psychological symptoms were within the normal range. Consistent with findings for heterosexual parents and their children, assessments of children's adjustment were significantly associated with measures of maternal mental health. These results underline the importance of maternal mental health as a predictor of children's adjustment among lesbian as well as among heterosexual families. *[Article copies available for a fee from The Haworth Document Delivery Service: 1-800-342-9678. E-mail address: <getinfo@haworthpressinc.com> Website: <http://www.HaworthPress.com> © 2001 by The Haworth Press, Inc. All rights reserved.]*

Normative research on lesbian mothers, gay fathers, and their children has generally reported that children growing up with lesbian and

Dr. Charlotte J. Patterson is affiliated with the Department of Psychology, 102 Gilmer Hall, University of Virginia, P.O. Box 400400, Charlottesville, VA 22904-4400 (E-mail: CJP@VIRGINIA.edu).

Support from the Society for Psychological Study of Social Issues for this work is gratefully acknowledged. Special thanks to Mitch Chyette, Deborah Cohn, Charlene Depner, Ellie Schindelman, and all of the participating families for their invaluable support and assistance. The author also wishes to thank Alicia Eddy, David Koppelman, Meg Michel, and Scott Spence for their efficient work in coding the data.

[Haworth co-indexing entry note]: "Families of the Lesbian Baby Boom: Maternal Mental Health and Child Adjustment." Patterson, Charlotte J. Co-published simultaneously in *Journal of Gay & Lesbian Psychotherapy* (The Haworth Medical Press, an imprint of The Haworth Press, Inc.) Vol. 4, No. 3/4, 2001, pp. 91-107; and: *Gay and Lesbian Parenting* (ed: Deborah F. Glazer, and Jack Drescher) The Haworth Medical Press, an imprint of The Haworth Press, Inc., 2001, pp. 91-107. Single or multiple copies of this article are available from The Haworth Document Delivery Service [1-800-342-9678, 9:00 a.m. - 5:00 p.m. (EST). E-mail address: getinfo@haworthpressinc.com].

gay parents are as well-adjusted as their peers growing up with hetero-sexual parents (Falk, 1989; Green & Bozett, 1991; Kirkpatrick, 1996; Laird, 1993; Patterson, 1992, 1997; Patterson & D'Augelli, 1998; Perrin, 1998; Tasker & Golombok, 1991, 1997). Little is yet known, however, about sources of individual differences among children of lesbian and gay families (Patterson, 1992; 1995-b). In homes headed by lesbian couples, one recent study found that mothers reported feel-ing more satisfied and children reported a greater sense of well-being when mothers shared the labor involved in childcare more evenly (Patterson, 1995-a). Another study reported similar findings for moth-ers, but not for children (Chan, Brooks, Raboy & Patterson, 1998), and much remains to be learned in this area. To explore the diversity among lesbian mother families, the present study was designed to examine sources of variation among lesbian mothers, considered as individuals, in contributing to mental health among their children.

Among the predictors of children's adjustment, maternal mental health plays an especially prominent role in the psychological research literature. Research on heterosexual families has shown that when mothers are psychologically healthy and well-adjusted, their children are also likely to develop in a positive fashion (Belsky, 1984; Belsky & Pensky, 1988; Miller, Cowan, Cowan, Hetherington & Clingem-peel, 1993). On the other hand, when mothers experience mental health problems such as depression or schizophrenia, their children are also more likely to experience difficulties (Downey & Coyne, 1990; Downey & Walker, 1992; Field, 1992; Gelfand & Teti, 1990). There-fore, factors that support maternal mental health may also be favorable for children's development. Although the existing research has fo-cused primarily on heterosexual families, one might expect that asso-ciations between maternal and child mental health would also occur in lesbian mother families.

Another factor often believed to influence children's adjustment is household composition (Garfinkel & McLanahan, 1986; McLanahan & Sandefur, 1994). The existing literature has revealed advantages accruing the children growing up in two-parent households, and has shown that these are due at least in part to differences in the economic situations of one- and two-parent homes (McLanahan & Sandefur, 1994). Thus, when economic stress is statistically controlled, the dif-ferences between children growing up in one- and two-parent homes become less pronounced (McLanahan & Sandefur, 1994).

Applied to lesbian families, mainstream research on household composition suggests that two-parent lesbian mother homes may be more likely than single lesbian mother homes to support favorable development among children. Indeed, on the basis of clinical impressions of lesbian families that she worked with, Kirkpatrick (1987) reported her impression that "children in households that included the mother's lesbian lover had a richer, more open and stable family life" (p. 204). On the basis of existing research, then, one might expect that children growing up in middle class two-parent lesbian-headed homes would be especially likely to show favorable development.

In contrast to expectations based on psychological research, the legal system in the United States has often operated on the basis of very different assumptions (Falk, 1989; Flaks, 1994; Patterson & Redding, 1996; Polikoff, 1986; Rivera, 1991). Judges have sometimes forbidden mothers to retain custody of minor children while living with lesbian partners; others have forbidden mothers from even so much as visiting overnight with their children in the presence of a lesbian partner (see Patterson & Redding, 1996). Such decisions would appear to reflect the view that whatever benefits a stable two-parent lesbian home might provide must be offset by the child's exposure to the mother's lesbian relationship, such that the net results for children in a two-parent lesbian home would be negative.

The present study was designed to evaluate contrasting expectations of psychological and (some) judicial traditions by assessing both maternal mental health and child adjustment among both one- and two-parent lesbian mother families. The sample was drawn from a group of families in which children had been born to or adopted early in life by lesbian mothers, i.e., from what have been called the "families of the lesbian baby boom" (Patterson, 1992; Lewin, 1993; Weston, 1991). Because the children had lived their entire lives in households headed by lesbian mothers, there was no possibility that results could be attributable to stresses associated with the break-up of a previous heterosexual family.

Studies of mental health among lesbian women have found lesbians to be very similar in their overall adjustment to matched groups of heterosexual women. Research has generally failed to reveal adjustment differences between lesbian and heterosexual samples of women, and both the American Psychiatric Association and the American Psychological Association have long rejected the notion that homosexuality per se represents any form of illness or disorder (Gonsiorek, 1991). Also, previous research based on the present sample of families (Patterson, 1994) revealed that children's overall development was proceeding normally. For example, children in this sample did not differ significantly on standardized assessments of social competence or behavior problems from national norms for representative samples of same-aged children (see Patterson, 1994). Thus, it was expected that the present sample of lesbian mothers would also show generally positive mental health.

Based on extrapolation from the literature on heterosexual families, it was expected that well-functioning mothers would be more likely to have well-adjusted children. Because of questions about the sources of reported advantages for children growing up in two-parent over those growing up in one-parent homes, the extent to which household composition would be a valuable predictor in this sample was left as an open question. Associations between maternal and child mental health were thus expected, but no predictions were made about possible associations of household composition with the other two variables among the relatively affluent lesbian mother families who took part in the present study.

METHOD

Participants

Eligibility and Recruitment. To be considered eligible, a family had to include at least one child between 4 and 9 years of age, who had been born to or adopted early in life by a lesbian mother or mothers. Due to practical constraints, the family also had to live within the greater San Francisco Bay Area. Any family that met these criteria was considered eligible to participate.

Recruitment began when the author contacted friends, acquaintances, and colleagues who might be likely to know eligible lesbian mother families. She described the research and asked help in locating families who might be willing to take part. She then contacted each potential family by telephone, explaining how she had obtained their name, describing the research, and asking whether they would be willing to participate. If a family agreed, an appointment was arranged for a visit to the family's home. The process of discussion, decision making, and appointment setting required a number of telephone calls in most cases, and in some cases, letters were also exchanged before an appointment was made. In all, contact was made with 39 eligible families, of whom 37 (95%) agreed to take part in the study.

Participating Families. Of the 37 participating families, 26 (70%) were headed by a lesbian couple and 7 (19%) were headed by a single mother living with her child or children. In the remaining 4 (11%) families, the child had been born to a lesbian couple who had since separated, and the child was in de facto joint custody (i.e., living part of the time with one mother and part of the time with the other mother). In this last group of families, one mother was out of town during the period of testing and so was not included in the study.

A total of 66 women took part in the study. Of these, 61 (92%) identified themselves as predominantly lesbian, and 5 (8%) identified themselves as predominantly bisexual. Their ages ranged from 28 to 53 years, with a mean age of 39.6 years. There were 61 (92%) self-described white or non-Hispanic Caucasian women, 2 (3%) African-American or black women, and 3 (4%) who described themselves as coming from other racial or ethnic backgrounds. Most were well-educated, employed outside the home, and relatively affluent (see Patterson, 1994 for details).

For the statistical analysis of data for this study, the biological or legal adoptive mother of the focal child was designated "Mother 1." If, as in most families, there was another mother, she was designated "Mother 2." No statement about the relative importance or behavior of either woman was intended by these labels; they were employed solely as a statistical convenience. In one family headed by a lesbian couple, the women did not wish to identify one as the biological and one as the nonbiological parent of the focal child; in this case, one was identified as Mother 1 and the other as Mother 2 by a coin toss.

In each family, the focal child was between 4 and 9 years of age (mean age: 6 years, 2 months); there were 19 girls and 18 boys. A total of 34 (92%) of the children were born to lesbian mothers, and 3 (8%) had been adopted by lesbian mothers. There were 30 (81%) children who were described by their mothers as white or non-Hispanic Caucasian, 3 (8%) as Hispanic, and 4 (11%) as another racial or ethnic heritage.

Materials

There were four principal assessments of adjustment. Mothers' adjustment was assessed using the Rosenberg Self-Esteem Scale and the

Derogatis Symptom Checklist. Children's adjustment was assessed using the Achenbach and Edelbrock Child Behavior Checklist, and with the Eder Children's Self-View Questionnaire. In addition, background information about the family was gathered in the context of a structured interview.

Mothers' Self-Esteem. Maternal self-esteem was assessed using the Rosenberg Self-Esteem Scale (Rosenberg, 1979). This scale consists of 10 statements, with four response alternatives, indicating the respondent's degree of agreement with each statement. Results were tabulated to obtain total scores, based upon the recommendations contained in Rosenberg (1979). Scores on this instrument can range from 0 to 6, with high scores indicating low levels of self-esteem.

Mothers' Symptoms. Maternal adjustment was assessed using the Derogatis Symptom Checklist–Revised (SCL-90-R; Derogatis, 1983), which consists of 90 items addressing a variety of psychological and somatic symptoms. Each respondent rated the extent to which she had been distressed by each symptom during the past week (0 = not at all, 4 = extremely). Test-retest reliability, internal consistency, and concurrent validity have all been shown to be adequate (Derogatis, 1983). Nine subscales (i.e., anger/hostility, anxiety, depression, interpersonal sensitivity, obsessive/compulsiveness, paranoid ideation, phobic anxiety, psychoticism, and somatization) were scored here, as well as a Global Severity Index which summarized the respondent's overall level of distress. Higher scores indicated greater distress.

Children's Social Competence and Behavior Problems. To assess both levels of child competence and child behavior problems, the Child Behavior Checklist (CBCL) (Achenbach & Edelbrock, 1983) was administered. The CBCL was selected because of its ability to identify both internalizing (e.g., inhibited or overcontrolled behavior) and externalizing (e.g., aggressive, antisocial, or undercontrolled behavior) problems as well as to assess levels of social competence. It is designed to be completed by parents. In this study, all participating mothers completed the instrument.

The CBCL is designed to record in a standardized format the competencies and behavior problems of children from 4 to 16 years of age (Achenbach & Edelbrock, 1983). There are 118 behavior problem items, and each one is scored on a three-point scale (not true, somewhat or sometimes true, very true or often true). Answers are tabulated to create subscales for internalizing, externalizing, and total behavior problems. The 20 social competence items assess an array of child competencies both at home and at school, and are tabulated to create a single score for social competence. Information about the reliability and validity of CBCL scores is available in Achenbach and Edelbrock (1983), and information about average scores for this sample of children is provided in Patterson (1994).

Children's Self-Concepts. Assessment of children's self-concepts was accomplished using 5 scales from Eder's (1990) Children's Self-View Questionnaire. These scales designed especially to assess psychological concepts of self among children from 3 to 8 years of age, assessed 5 different dimensions of children's views of themselves (i.e., aggression, social closeness, social potency, stress reaction, and well-being). Using hand puppets, the CSVQ was administered individually to participating children. Their answers were tape-recorded for later scoring according to the recommendations contained in Eder (1990). Information on reliability and validity of these scales is given in Eder (1990), and information about average scores for the present sample of children can be found in Patterson (1994).

Interviews

As described above, an appointment was arranged for the author to visit each family's home. When the researcher arrived at the home, she explained the study, answered questions, and asked for written consent from the mother or mothers who were present; oral assent was also obtained from children. The visit began with a semistructured family interview, which involved a number of questions about family background (e.g., maternal education and occupation) and family history (e.g., circumstances surrounding the focal child's birth or adoption). This was followed by an individual interview with the focal child, which included Eder's Children's Self-View Questionnaire (Patterson, 1994). During the time that the interviewer was with the focal child, mothers were asked to fill out a number of questionnaires, among which were the Rosenberg Self-Esteem Scale, the Derogatis SCL-90, and the Achenbach and Edelbrock CBCL. In families headed by a lesbian couple, the women were asked to complete the questionnaires without consulting one another. When both mothers and children had completed these materials, they were thanked for their assistance and given an opportunity to ask any questions about the study. Each visit lasted between 90 and 150 minutes.

RESULTS

Normative results for maternal adjustment are presented first. Because the normative results for children's adjustment have been reported elsewhere (Patterson, 1994), they are not described in any detail here. However, in an effort to locate sources of individual differences in children's adjustment, maternal and child adjustment are examined as a function of household composition (i.e., one- versus two-parent households). Finally, the extent to which maternal mental health is a predictor of children's adjustment is also examined.

Maternal Self-Esteem and Symptoms

Total scores on the Rosenberg Self-Esteem Scale were calculated for each mother, following the method described by Rosenberg (1979), and the resulting mean scores are shown in Table 1. As can be seen in the table, the means for Mother 1 and Mother 2 were almost identical, and both were well within the range of normal functioning. These results indicate that lesbian mothers who took part in this research reported generally positive views about themselves.

For the Derogatis SCL-90, nine subscale scores and one global severity index (GSI) were computed for each mother, and average scores on each measure were calculated both for Mother 1 and for Mother 2. The average subscale scores and T scores for each subscale and for the GSI are shown in Table 1. T scores are based on the norms of female non-patient samples contained in Derogatis (1983).

As can be seen in Table 1, mean scores for Mother 1 and for Mother 2 were virtually identical for most subscales as well as for the GSI, and they were all well within a normal range. None of the T scores deviates substantially (i.e., more than one standard deviation) from the expected mean of 50, indicating that lesbian mothers' reports of symptoms were no greater and no smaller than those expected for any other group of women of the same age. Thus, like the findings for adjustment of children in this sample (Patterson, 1994), those for maternal adjustment revealed that lesbian mothers who took part in this study reported good psychological adjustment.

Household Composition, Mothers' Symptoms and Children's Adjustment

It was also of interest to evaluate the extent to which the adjustment of children and their mothers might be linked to household composi-

TABLE 1. Means and T-scores of SCL-90-R Subscales and Rosenberg Self-Esteem Scale for Biological and Non-Biological Mothers

	Biological Mothers		Non-Biological Mothers	
	Mean	T-score[1]	Mean	T-score
SCL-90-R subscales				
Anger/hostility	.36	55	.31	52
Anxiety	.29	52	.24	51
Depression	.40	53	.43	53
Interpersonal sensitivity	.33	53	.36	54
Obsessive/compulsiveness	.31	50	.51	54
Paranoid ideation	.32	52	.25	52
Phobic anxiety	.01	44	.12	53
Psychoticism	.11	53	.11	53
Somatization	.29	50	.32	50
Global Severity Index (GSI)	.34	53	.38	55
Rosenberg Self-Esteem	2.49		2.58	

[1]T-scores based on norms of non-patient group according to Derogatis (1983); T-scores for Rosenberg scale were not available.

tion. In particular, it was desirable to assess whether children were in better psychological health when mothers were living with lesbian partners (as one might predict based on research with heterosexual families) or (as the legal system has sometimes maintained) whether they were better off when mothers were living alone with their child or children (i.e., without a lesbian partner in the home).

To address these questions, the sample was divided into two-parent households (i.e., families that were headed by two lesbian mothers who lived together in the same household; $n = 26$ families), and one-parent households (i.e., all other families in the sample; $n = 11$ families), and adjustment scores for the two groups were compared. The results revealed that mothers' self-esteem did not vary as a function of household composition, nor did mothers' overall psychosocial adjustment, as measured by the SCL-90 GSI (both t's < 1). Children in one-parent households were *not* described as having more behavior problems overall than those in two-parent households, $t (11, 24) = 1.17$, n.s. There were no differences in any of the 5 child self-concept scales as a function of household composition (all t's < 1). Thus, household composition was not associated with adjustment among mothers or their children in this sample.

Associations Between Maternal and Child Adjustment

The degree to which variations in maternal and child adjustment were associated with one another was also explored. Both mothers' and children's scores on assessments of adjustment were within the normal range, but some variability was nevertheless evident among individuals. To evaluate whether the variability in children's scores was predictable from knowledge of the variability in mothers' scores, associations between the two sets of variables were examined.

Results showed that mothers who reported experiencing more symptoms themselves were also likely to report more behavior problems among their children. Regression analyses testing the four principal indicators of maternal well-being (viz., GSI and self-esteem scores for both mothers) as predictors of child behavior problems revealed that both mothers' reports of symptoms were significantly related to Mother 1's reports of children's total behavior problems, F (4, 32) = 3.31, p < .05, accounting together for 23% of the variance. The zero-order Pearson correlations were .39 for Mother 1's GSI scores and .16 for Mother 2's GSI scores. Rosenberg self-esteem scores did not add significantly to these predictions, nor were there any significant predictors of any of the five self-concept scales for children. Among the group of lesbian families we studied, then, assessments of maternal mental health were associated with their ratings of children's adjustment.

In an effort to locate more precisely the aspects of maternal mental health that were associated with reports about children's behavior, each of the subscale scores of the SCL-90 was also examined. Table 2 shows the zero-order correlations between SCL-90 subscale scores and reported behavior problems separately for Mother 1 and for Mother 2. For Mother 1, 3 of the 9 subscales–anger/hostility, r = .36, p < .05, depression, r =.52, p < .01, and obsessive-compulsiveness, r = .45, p < .01–as well as the global severity index, r = .39, p < .05, were significantly correlated with children's total behavior problems. For Mother 2, the GSI score was not significantly associated with her report of children's behavior problems when considered alone, so individual subscale scores were not interpreted. Overall, then, biological mothers who reported more symptoms also reported that their children evidenced more behavior problems; the symptoms that differentiated among child outcomes were those associated with anger, hostility, depression, difficulty concentrating, and problems with decision-making.

DISCUSSION

Consistent with the findings of a substantial body of research on heterosexual families, our findings revealed that well-adjusted lesbian mothers were more likely than those suffering from even moderate psychological symptoms to report that their children are themselves developing in a positive fashion. Lesbian mothers in this sample generally described both themselves and their children as well-adjusted, so the range of scores was relatively small. Even within the restricted range of scores studied here, however, assessments of maternal mental health were distinctly more important than household composition in

TABLE 2. Correlations of Biological and Non-Biological Mothers' Symptoms and Self-Esteem with Child's Total Behavior Problem Scores According to That Mother

	Biological Mothers	Non-Biological Mothers
SCL-90-R Subscales		
Anger/hostility	.36*	.41*
Anxiety	.16	.10
Depression	.52**	.30
Interpersonal sensitivity	.30	.14
Obsessive/compulsiveness	.45**	.22
Paranoid ideation	.31	.45*
Phobic anxiety	.05	−.17
Psychoticism	.17	.19
Somatization	.11	.19
Global Severity Index (GSI)	.39*	.16
Rosenberg Self-Esteem	.23	.25

Note. The correlation between both mothers' observations of total behavior problems, in families with two mothers, was $r = .48$, $p < .01$. For biological mothers, n = 37; for non-biological mothers, n = 26.
* $p < .05$; ** $p < .01$

predicting outcomes for children. These results are thus consistent with the notion that factors favoring maternal mental health may also favor the psychosocial development of children (Belsky, 1984; Belsky & Pensky, 1988; Miller et al., 1993).

The first major result was that lesbian mothers in this sample reported few symptoms, and good overall mental health. Consistent with the considerable literature on mental health of lesbian women (Gonsiorek, 1991), results showed that both maternal self-esteem and maternal reports of symptoms were in the normal range of scores expected for women in this age range (Derogatis, 1983; Rosenberg, 1979). While consistent with reports about mental health of divorced lesbian mothers that comprise the existing literature (Patterson, 1997), these results are the first to focus on mental health among women who have chosen motherhood after assuming lesbian identities. The findings also revealed no differences between biological and nonbiological lesbian mothers in this regard; both scored in the normal range on our assessments of mental health.

The second major finding was that children's adjustment did not differ significantly as a function of household composition. Although much of the literature on children growing up in heterosexual families has suggested that children in one-parent homes are at a disadvantage, differences between children in one-parent and two-parent households did not approach statistical significance in this sample. As in the literature on heterosexual families, one-parent families in the present sample did report lower incomes, t (35) = 3.05, $p < .01$, but even the lower incomes of one-parent lesbian families studied here, averaging about $30,000-$50,000 per year, placed them in relatively comfortable financial circumstances. In contrast, incomes in one-parent heterosexual households are generally lower, and many of the disadvantages suffered by children in one-parent heterosexual households can be attributed to family economic stress (McLanahan & Sandefur, 1994). Whether for this or for other reasons, household composition was not a strong predictor of child adjustment among lesbian families studied here. Overall, as reported in more detail elsewhere (Patterson, 1994, 1997), children were well-adjusted.

The third major finding was that, even within the relatively restricted range of scores studied here, there were significant associations between maternal mental health and children's adjustment. Even though maternal and child mental health were both generally good, biological mothers' reports of symptoms were still significantly related to children's behavior problems, as assessed here. Given that biological mothers in this sample were more likely than non-biological mothers to be responsible for childcare (Patterson, 1995-a), it is not surprising that children's adjustment would be more closely tied to reports of the mental health of biological than to non-biological mothers. Consistent with the findings of research on heterosexual families, our findings serve to underline the importance of maternal mental health for children's adjustment.

At the same time as these findings add to existing knowledge about the families of the lesbian baby boom, they also demonstrate the generality of findings from earlier research on heterosexual families. Although earlier studies have reported both normative and individual differences findings about lesbian families (Patterson, 1997), this is the first study to report on self-esteem and symptoms among mothers of the lesbian baby boom, and it is the first to examine household composition and maternal mental health as predictors of child outcomes in these families. As has been evident in recent studies of heterosexual and lesbian families (Chan, Raboy & Patterson, 1998), these findings suggest the significance of family process (e.g., family conflict) over that of family structure (e.g., one- versus two-parent households) in affecting child outcomes. To provide further information about these issues, future research should be designed to include variables relevant both to structure and to process.

From the standpoint of the legal system, the current findings suggest that the best interests of children in lesbian families may be served by interventions that have a positive impact on maternal mental health, but they provide no evidence in favor of interventions aimed at influencing household composition. The results did not suggest that children would be better off in single-parent lesbian households such as those sometimes stipulated by the courts; in fact, household composition was unrelated to children's adjustment among the families studied here. Assessments of maternal mental health, in contrast, were significant predictors of outcomes for children. Although preliminary in nature, the current findings thus can be interpreted to suggest that judges who wish to maximize the best interests of children in custody disputes involving lesbian mothers should focus attention not on household composition as such but rather on conditions that are associated with maternal mental health (Patterson & Redding, 1996).

Although the current findings have much to offer, they also are characterized by a number of limitations that should be acknowledged. The group of lesbian mother families studied here was a sample of convenience, drawn from a single geographical area. The mothers who participated in the study were predominantly white, well-educated and relatively affluent. Given practical constraints, it was not possible to collect observational data, nor to gain access to informants outside the families themselves. Both assessments of mothers' and children's adjustment were provided by maternal reports, and some method variance was thus held in common between assessments of the two categories of variables. These and other limitations of the present research suggest that our findings are best regarded as preliminary results, in need of further evaluation among larger and more diverse samples, using a broader array of informants and assessment procedures, over more occasions of measurement (Patterson, 1997).

It is particularly important to acknowledge the possible role of rater biases in contributing to the associations between assessments of maternal and child mental health. Because significant associations were found between maternal mental health and children's adjustment only when both were rated by mothers, the possibility of rater bias must be considered. Research with heterosexual families has also encountered this possibility (Compas, Phares, Banez & Howell, 1991) and, in the case of associations between marital quality and children's adjustment, rater bias has sometimes been found to be responsible for an important share of the observed associations (e.g., McHale, Freitag, Crouter & Bartko, 1991). On the other hand, the idea that depressed mothers provide negatively biased reports about their children's adjustment has been found to be without empirical foundation (Richters, 1992), and the issue remains unsettled. In future research, it would be valuable to obtain data about both maternal and child functioning from multiple sources so that possible rater biases could be evaluated in a systematic fashion.

In summary, this study examined associations between maternal and child adjustment among a sample of the families of the lesbian baby boom. Consistent with expectations (Falk, 1989; Gonsiorek, 1991; Patterson, 1992, 1997), scores for both maternal and child adjustment fell within the normal range. Although neither mothers nor children living in one-parent households differed in their overall adjustment from those living in two-parent households, there were consistent associations between variations in maternal mental health and those in child adjustment. Even within the restricted range of scores studied here, mothers who described their own adjustment in positive terms were also likely to report that their children were developing well. Overall, the results contribute to an appreciation of diversity among the families of the lesbian baby boom and, more generally, also add to understanding of the role of sexual orientation in human development (Patterson, 1995-c; Patterson & D'Augelli, 1998).

REFERENCES

Achenbach, T. M., & Edelbrock, C. (1983). *Manual for the Child Behavior Checklist and Revised Child Behavior Profile*. Burlington VT: University of Vermont, Department of Psychiatry.

Belsky, J. (1984). The determinants of parenting: A process model. *Child Development, 55*, 83-96.

Belsky, J. & Pensky, E. (1988). Developmental history, personality, and family relationships: Toward an emergent family system. In R. A. Hinde & J. Stevenson-Hinde (Eds.), *Relationships within families: Mutual influences* (pp. 193-217). Oxford, England: Oxford University Press.

Chan, R. W., Raboy, B., & Patterson, C. J. (1998-a). Psychosocial adjustment among children conceived via donor insemination by lesbian and heterosexual mothers. *Child Development, 69*, 443-457.

Chan, R. W., Brooks, R. C., Raboy, B., & Patterson, C. J. (1998-b). Division of labor among lesbian and heterosexual parents: Associations with children's adjustment. *Journal of Family Psychology, 12*, 402-419.

Compas, B. E., Phares, V., Banez, G. A., & Howell, D. C. (1991). Correlates of internalizing and externalizing behavior problems: Perceived competence, causal attributions, and parental symptoms. *Journal of Abnormal Child Psychology, 19*, 197-218.

Derogatis, L. R. (1983). *SCL-90-R administration, scoring, and procedures manual*. Towson MD: Clinical Psychometric Research.

Downey, G. & Coyne, J. C. (1990). Children of depressed parents: An integrative review. *Psychological Bulletin, 108*, 50-76.

Downey, G. & Walker, E. (1992). Distinguishing family-level and child-level influences on the development of depression and aggression in children at risk. *Development and Psychopathology, 4*, 81-95.

Eder, R. A. (1990). Uncovering young children's psychological selves: Individual and developmental differences. *Child Development, 61*, 849-863.

Falk, P. J. (1989). Lesbian mothers: Psychosocial assumptions in family law. *American Psychologist, 44*, 941-947.

Field, T. (1992). Infants of depressed mothers. *Development and Psychopathology, 4*, 49-66.

Flaks, D. (1994). Gay and lesbian families: Judicial assumptions, scientific realities. *William and Mary Bill of Rights Journal, 3*, 345-372.

Garfinkel, I., & McLanahan, S. (1986). *Single mothers and their children: A new American dilemma*. Washington, DC: The Urban Institute Press.

Gelfand, D. M. & Teti, D. M. (1990). Effects of maternal depression on children. *Clinical Psychology Review, 10*, 329-353.

Gonsiorek, J. (1991). The empirical basis for the demise of the illness model of homosexuality. In J. C. Gonsiorek & J. D. Weinrich (Eds.), *Homosexuality: Research implications for public policy* (pp. 115-136). Newbury Park, CA: Sage.

Green, G. D., & Bozett, F. W. (1991). Lesbian mothers and gay fathers. In J. C. Gonsiorek & J. D. Weinrich (Eds.), *Homosexuality: Research implications for public policy* (pp. 197-214). Newbury Park, CA: Sage.

Kirkpatrick, M. (1987). Clinical implications of lesbian mother studies. *Journal of Homosexuality, 14*, 201-211.

Kirkpatrick, M. (1996). Lesbians as parents. In R. P. Cabaj & T. S. Stein (Eds.), *Textbook of homosexuality and mental health*. Washington, DC: American Psychiatric Press, Inc.

Laird, J. (1993). Lesbian and gay families. In F. Walsh (Ed.), *Normal family processes* (2nd ed., pp. 282-328). New York: Guilford.

Lewin, E. (1993). *Lesbian mothers: Accounts of gender in American culture*. Ithaca, NY: Cornell University Press.

McHale, S. M., Freitag, M. K., Crouter, A. C. & Bartko, W. T. (1991). Connections between dimensions of marital quality and school-age children's adjustment. *Journal of Applied Developmental Psychology, 12*, 1-17.

McLanahan, S., & Sandefur, G. (1994). *Growing up with a single parent: What hurts, what helps*. Cambridge, MA: Harvard University Press.

Miller, N. B., Cowan, P. A., Cowan, C. P., Hetherington, E. M., & Clingempeel, W. G. (1993). Externalizing in preschoolers and early adolescents: A cross-study replication of a family model. *Developmental Psychology, 29*, 3-18.

Patterson, C. J. (1992). Children of lesbian and gay parents. *Child Development, 63*, 1025-1042.

Patterson, C. J. (1994). Children of the lesbian baby boom: Behavioral adjustment, self-concepts, and sex-role identity. In B. Greene & G. Herek (Eds.), *Contemporary Perspectives on Lesbian and Gay Psychology: Theory, Research, and Application* (pp. 156-175). Beverly Hills, CA: Sage.

Patterson, C. J. (1995-a). Families of the lesbian baby boom: Parents' division of labor and children's adjustment. *Developmental Psychology, 31*, 115-123.

Patterson, C. J. (1995-b). Lesbian mothers, gay fathers, and their children. In A. R. D'Augelli & C. J. Patterson (Eds.), *Lesbian, Gay and Bisexual Identities Over the Lifespan: Psychological Perspectives* (pp. 262-290). New York: Oxford University Press.

Patterson, C. J. (1995-c). Sexual orientation and human development: An overview. *Developmental Psychology, 31*, 3-11.

Patterson, C. J. (1997). Children of lesbian and gay parents. In T. Ollendick & R. Prinz (Eds.), *Advances in Clinical Child Psychology*, Vol. 19. New York: Plenum Press.

Patterson, C. J., & D'Augelli, A. R. (Eds.). (1998). *Lesbian, Gay and Bisexual Identities in Families*. New York: Oxford University Press.

Patterson, C. J., & Redding, R. (1996). Lesbian and gay families with children: Public policy implications of social science research. *Journal of Social Issues, 52,* 29-50.

Perrin, E. C. (1998). Children whose parents are lesbian or gay. *Contemporary Pediatrics, 15,* 113-130.

Polikoff, N. (1986). Lesbian mothers, lesbian families, legal obstacles, legal challenges. *Review of Law and Social Change, 14,* 907-914.

Richters, J. E. (1992). Depressed mothers as informants about their children: A critical review of the evidence for distortion. *Psychological Bulletin, 112,* 485-499.

Rivera, R. R. (1991). Sexual orientation and the law. In J. C. Gonsiorek & J. D. Weinrich (Eds.), *Homosexuality: Research implications for public policy* (pp. 81-100). Newbury Park, CA: Sage Publications.

Rosenberg, S. (1979). *Conceiving the self.* New York: Basic Books.

Tasker, F. & Golombok, S. (1991). Children raised by lesbian mothers: The empirical evidence. *Family Law, 21,* 184-187.

Tasker, F. L. & Golombok, S. (1997). *Growing up in a lesbian family: Effects on child development.* New York: Guilford.

Weston, K. (1991). *Families we choose: Lesbians, gays, kinship.* New York: Columbia University Press.

Excerpts
from *The Velveteen Father:*
An Unexpected Journey
to Parenthood

Jesse Green

I

This first excerpt from *The Velveteen Father* is taken from Part I of the book, which chronicles the attempts of Green's partner Andy to father a child long before the two men met. Andy initially wants a child who is biologically related to him. This leads to a series of attempts at helping a lesbian couple get pregnant via alternative insemination. When the couple ultimately rejects him as a donor, Andy must face the previously-rejected prospect of adopting a child. Here, Green muses on the unfairness of reproductive biology and explores some of the prejudices surrounding adoption:

[Andy's] experience with alternative insemination was far from atypical. It seemed, upon closer examination, that this procedure led in most cases to one of two outcomes: failure and acrimony or success

Jesse Green is a much-anthologized, award-winning journalist whose articles appear regularly in *The New York Times Magazine* as well as in *The New Yorker, The Washington Post, New York, Premiere, The Yale Review, GQ, Philadelphia, Out, Mirabella, Elle,* and *Parenting.* He is also the author of a novel, *O Beautiful,* and numerous short stories and essays (E-mail: Jesse1958@aol.com).

[Haworth co-indexing entry note]: "Excerpts from *The Velveteen Father: An Unexpected Journey to Parenthood.*" Green, Jesse. Co-published simultaneously in *Journal of Gay & Lesbian Psychotherapy* (The Haworth Medical Press, an imprint of The Haworth Press, Inc.) Vol. 4, No. 3/4, 2001, pp. 109-118; and: *Gay and Lesbian Parenting* (ed: Deborah F. Glazer, and Jack Drescher) The Haworth Medical Press, an imprint of The Haworth Press, Inc., 2001, pp. 109-118.

and acrimony. Contractual obligations were as unlikely to produce happy results in the manufacture of babies as they were in custody cases later, and the geometry of the lesbian couple at two points of the triangle with the lone sperm donor at the third enforced certain inequities. The inequities were at base biological, of course. The one thing a man lacked in order to give birth to a child was so vast and mysterious that religions were built around it; a woman only lacked a teaspoonful of something men wasted by the gallon. This gave the whole production an unsavory black widow-meets-D. H. Lawrence odor: Come and then die. The putatively virile man so central to the process was actually in the women's employ: a hired hand, as it were.

Is it disloyal of me to surmise that Andy contributed to the disaster, if only through a lack of self-knowledge? Looking at him now, I don't think he could have been happy with the arrangement, even if it had somehow worked out. What he wanted out of fathering a child was more than would be likely to result from vacation visits and paying for college. Unfortunately, he knew less about what he wanted than about what he *didn't* want. He didn't want (for instance) to get involved with any more contractual masturbation schemes. He didn't, of course, want a dishonest marriage: It was hard to say who was saddest in such ménages, the sneaking husband, the unfulfilled wife, or the anxious children. And yet Andy had somehow come to believe that he didn't want to adopt a baby, either. It's hard now to credit his reasoning: that babies should be breast-fed and that an adopted newborn, dependent on a bottle, was cruelly deprived of an important, perhaps a crucial, experience. "Something about immunity," he now mutters in defense of that position. "Immunity was in the air."

All due respect to the breast; it's a wonderful organ and undoubtedly a more esthetically pleasing vending system for nourishment than latex nipples and presterilized liners in plastic bottles with teddy bear designs. But a distaste for the bottle could only have been covering some other, more substantial distaste. Was the antiadoption prejudice of previous generations reasserting itself? Andy's mother, who had breast-fed her two sons, seemed to have felt that adoption, with its bottle feedings, was deeply unnatural: not direct and biological like the flow of milk from mother to newborn, but disjoint, synthetic–an abstract formula. The liquid involved was even *called* formula, which seemed to suggest all sorts of potentially mathematical exertions.

Andy had never been good at math, but he'd loved mythology, and mythology (see Oedipus) did not speak well of adoption.

Even my mother and father, mild and liberal though they are, permitted themselves this casual bigotry. Little spoken of except as slander, adoption was vaguely understood in my house as a procedure occasioned by a physical defect in the parents–infertility, a lack of robustness–and prefiguring emotional defects in the children. The fact that emotional defects were rampant among the biological offspring of their friends and acquaintances did not seem to threaten the connection they made between stranger and strangeness, for ancient clan issues were involved here. Perhaps especially among the descendants of Moses (himself adopted, by Pharaoh's daughter) the distinction between insider and outsider, and thus the legibility of bloodlines, became a talisman of safety in an unsafe world. Which is why none but the most fanatical Lubavitcher sects proselytize; to the contrary: In the game of "Is It Good for the Jews?" (Einstein, yes; Roy Cohn, no) it was often noted with an asterisk of relief that psychopaths like David "Son of Sam" Berkowitz turned out to have been landsmen only by accident–that is, by adoption.

In such an environment, the only thing more unnatural than a couple choosing adoption would be a man choosing adoption on his own. As a source of passion–the kind of passion mothers are admired for possessing and vilified for lacking–fatherhood, even biological fatherhood, was suspicious. Women needed to have children to be seen as normal and fulfilled, but too much childlust in a man made him a freak: a possible pedophile, or at least homosexual. What are we to make of those fathers who, desperately wanting to nurse their own babies, convince quack doctors to inject them with hormones? We think them ridiculous, perhaps disgusting, especially since the halfhearted lactation thus stimulated could not nourish a guinea pig. The pleasure, if any, derived by the man–ah, pleasure, that American criminal–seals the sin, though the pleasures of female breast-feeding are tolerated as an unavoidable side effect of biology. A man who wants to adopt a child is often seen in a similar role: stealing from a woman the one thing society allows (indeed forces) her to keep for herself. Was it finally unnatural–that is, unhealthy–for a man to raise a child without a woman? Was it *selfish?*

On the other hand, if the television of my youth was to be believed, many men–widowers, that is–raised children alone, although they had a habit of hiring nannies whom they later married. Other TV dads fell in love with widows and adopted their brood, raising the kids (the phrase went) *as their own.* The unspoken anxiety to which these youthful deaths and family reconfigurations alluded was divorce, which by 1965 was beginning its Sherman's march through the American familyland. In its opaque and syrupy story lines, television was answering the question of what to do with the kids displaced by the fires along the way. Blend them, merge them, fold them into the corporation–a subtext that spoke to the underlying scariness of an unclaimed child. Adoption seemed to challenge the ownership fixations (and the anxieties beneath those fixations) of a postwar American consumer society whose icon of successful adulthood was a paid-off mortgage. Who really owned an adopted child? It was never asked who really owned the other kind.

II

In the second section of *The Velveteen Father,* entitled "The Tear Beat," Green delves into his own history, from his Philadelphia childhood to his New York career in journalism. Much of that journalism has been about the AIDS epidemic, and a repeated theme in his published accounts was that of the mother who loses a child. The moving story of the "crybaby" is one of four times in the book when Green interrupts his nonfiction narrative to present fairy-tale-like sections that present and comment upon the issues from a different perspective:

Once upon a time there was a kingdom that had no salt. It was landlocked, so there was no sea to provide it, and not even the elders remembered anymore the location of the caves from which the crystals had, in ancient times, been mined. Salt, however, was crucial to the people's health; without it they fell into stuporous trances, and no work (or too much work) got done. Those who were wealthy enough imported their supply, at great expense, from realms beyond the desert; but the trading routes were dangerous, lined with bones and thieves. Everyone else made do by swallowing their tears, except that–and here was the heart of the problem–most of them, once they were older than five, could not remember how to cry.

In this kingdom, a certain kind of child was therefore prized. He was called a crybaby–not because he cried so much himself (he did) but because he was able to get others to do so. A baby thought to possess this power was a source of pride to his family, for the custom of the kingdom was that, in return for his services, he would be paid a tithe from any tears he elicited. A very talented crybaby could net a vial a day, which he brought home to be sealed under wax in blue glass goblets until needed.

But if he was a source of pride, he was also a source of worry; he had always to be protected from the threat of kidnapping, for there was such a black market in tears. It was necessary to send him to expensive schools, run by a faculty of aged basset hounds, to learn the secret methods. Nor was the crybaby especially easy to live with. He had overly firm opinions. He ate peculiarly. He doubted himself and was sure of himself at exactly the wrong moments, and so was impossible to comfort. In short, he was odd and arrogant and glowed with intent, which many admired but most shied away from. People are afraid of the radiant child. And so is the child himself.

One crybaby or another was always being hailed as especially effective. His teachers would admire his particular style in poking his stick, or insinuating his needle, or patting a mother's hair just behind her ears–mothers' tears were deemed the most potent. His skills were so great that eventually the elders, in consultation with the faculty of bassets, would send him on a dangerous journey. Provided with only a faded map and a sad book about a spider, the boy was sent off into the desert in search of the ancient salt mines. "Follow your heart," his mother would tell him. "And the vultures," would say his father.

For many years no one knew what happened to these boys, for none of them ever returned. Until . . .

One night, a mother was awakened by a noise in her kitchen. There, having a glass of milk, sat her son.

"Did you find the mines?" she breathlessly asked.

"Yes," he said, "but they were empty."

"Oh. But did you find anything else?"

"Yes: the boys–I call them boys, for none has aged–living in the empty caves."

"But how do they survive?"

"They make each other cry with their stories and swallow each other's tears."

"And why did you, alone among them, choose to return?"

"No: They all returned, just as I have, to see their mothers. They

stayed one night but then went back to the empty caves. And there they remained. If you never knew, it was only because none of the mothers dared speak of it. Perhaps that way it still seemed possible–"

"I will speak of it," said his mother defiantly, but then stopped cold. "Will you go back?"

He looked at her, and started crying. By force of habit, he drew out a vial to catch the drops.

III

In the third section of *The Velveteen Father,* as he and Andy are beginning their relationship, Green, here still a single gay man, muses on the sights, sounds, and smells of childrearing:

Back in college, I tortured one of my best friends by describing what he would be like at forty; the idea of being forty was torture enough, but I cruelly embellished the portrait with Suburban Gothic details. He would have, I told him, a schoolteacher spouse, an adorable child, a receding hairline, and a wood-paneled Estate Wagon. To a twenty-year-old rebel with esthetic aspirations, this was tantamount to saying he would die in a hole with his Shriner's cap on. Not to worry for Michael, though: As it turned out, I was precise but not accurate. At thirty-seven, it looked as if I was the one who'd be ending up with the schoolteacher spouse (well, a guidance counselor), the receding hairline, and (in a way) the adorable child. Whereas Michael, though at least he was almost totally bald, was appearing off-Broadway as an East German transsexual rock diva while moonlighting on guitar with a post-punk band and serially dating leggy blondes.

At least I didn't have the Estate Wagon. I had never owned an automobile, and doubted I ever would. For the price of garaging in New York City, you could buy an extra set of internal organs. If you didn't garage, you were courting theft, not to mention subjecting yourself to the insane calculus of New York's parking regulations. Best to rent when you needed a ride: Was that not my grand philosophy? But then, in the week after his mother died, Andy finally traded in what was left of his Lancer and, hocking part of his Board of Education pension, bought a new car. Or was it a car? It was a huge gleaming thing, a silver bullet, aerodynamic and all kitted out with velour and cupholders and integrated child seats. Two integrated child seats.

We called the van the Space Station Mir and wondered how it would ever get filled. Andy imagined Boy Scout troops and Hebrew school car pools and platters of cupcakes for PTA bake sales. I imagined it just as it was the first time I saw it: clean and empty. God knows, the rest of my life with Andy looked as if it would be messy and full; here was something new, with no history, no mark of other lives upon it. And look: There was even a place to store coins! For all my antisuburban rhetoric I was bourgeois enough to love its luxurious thingness: the way it perfectly accomplished what it was supposed to be. The day Andy brought it home, we just sat in it for a few minutes and sniffed. It would not have that nice, new smell for long.

We'd had six dates in one month by then (if you include packing up his late mother's apartment as a date) and had decided to spend our first weekend together at Andy's little house on Long Island. At noon on a Friday in early July, we therefore loaded our luggage into the maw of the space station and set out on our maiden voyage. Erez, strapped into one of the fold-out child seats, sucked on a bottle and looked happily around. Chauncey the dog lay on the floor beside him. As we merged onto the Long Island Expressway, the car's digital compass correctly told us we were heading east: We all but applauded.

I did not take it as an ill omen when Chauncey tried to snatch my biscotti. I already knew that Andy's theory of dog-rearing (if not child-rearing) involved plenty of love and very little food. He seemed to think there was a fixed sum of kibble in a dog's lifetime; feed him less and he would live longer. It is true that Chauncey never got fat and was hale and athletic at nearly fourteen. But it is also true that he was constantly ravenous. His bowl, when put before him, was empty in seconds. The rest of the time he nudged around and begged under the table and sucked up every fallen scrap of Erez's meals like a vacuum cleaner. Andy liked that.

We drove along happily for the first half-hour. Then Erez started to make funny noises. I had heard the term "projectile vomit" before but never witnessed it. I'm sure you could do intricate calculations involving the speed of the car and the force of the retch to determine the maximum curdal displacement. What I can tell you is that pretty much the entire right side of the cabin was covered. And then, hungry Chauncey began to chow down. Erez giggled.

I was stunned but stalwart. After stopping at a roadside market to buy paper towels and Evian (they would not give us anything to clean up with), we wiped down Erez and what we could of the car and set off again with all the windows and the sun roof open. Soon Erez started making odd noises again–this time from the left child seat, the right one having become so encrusted with vomit it would not lock properly. "Oh no!" I shouted, and covered my face. But he did not vomit. How can I describe what happened now? Perhaps all the previous excitement had dislodged Erez's diaper–or perhaps the devil had possessed his bowels. In any case I looked over my shoulder in horror as a steady stream of brown sludge extruded itself from Erez's shorts. It did not stop. It never stopped. Erez giggled as hungry Chauncey began to chow down.

"I guess the car is christened," said Andy, patting my dead cold hand.

I guess I was, too. But even if I didn't yet have a sense of what was in store for me, I would very soon, for the morning after our arrival at Andy's house Erez promptly began to teethe. The beautiful child was hot with pain, whimpering and then screaming like a bright red kettle; nothing would soothe him except Andy's shoulder. But what would soothe me? It wasn't just the noise, though that was terrible; it was not knowing–not ever being able to know–what the crying wanted. I stood before the tortured baby, helpless as when a tourist asks directions in an impenetrably foreign language.

A child's miseries, like his colds (as I'd soon learn), are highly contagious, and I proved susceptible. Andy, on the other hand, seemed to be buoyed by Erez's wretchedness, or at least not sunk by it; it gave him a clarity of purpose that was otherwise elusive. His entire life's work in that moment was solely to be a comfort to his son, and there was no one on earth who could do the job better. It wasn't that he knew any magic words to chant; he didn't say much at all, out loud. It's that he remained cheerful and calm, unfazed by the assault of such huge unhappiness. This was part of his imperfectionism: He could tolerate and even thrive on disruption and disarray. Was there a more useful quality for a father to have in moments like this? Whereas I was a zombie, suffering from some sort of empathy disorder: My teeth started hurting. I thought I might cry.

IV

In the fourth and final section of the book, after Andy adopts their second child Lucas, Green invites his readers to a gender-bending bris (Jewish ritual circumcision):

"May the one who comes be blessed": Thus began the circumcision service two days later. Sixty people crowded into Andy's apartment for the noon affair, including dozens of delegates from Andy's rangy family and three from mine: my mother, father, and nephew. All were kind enough, upon arriving, not to mention that we looked wooden and sallow, with raccoon rings around our eyes; we had barely slept since the boy arrived forty hours before, and our hearts (I could feel Andy's, too) were clanking, loud and irregular, like the radiators.

At least the baby was getting cuter; what sleep we had lost, he had found and kept. His capuchin face had begun to unfold, his redness to recede. Everyone admired his sequin eyes: Is he Chinese? they asked.

"No, Jewish," I inevitably said. "As you will see."

Not *all* would see. We hired a sitter to keep Erez and my nephew busy in the nursery during the circumcision itself; if we had made our peace with the implications of the surgery on the baby, we were not so sure of its effect on a toddler who might catch a glimpse. Probably we should have hired a sitter for the adult men, too. They visibly blanched as the mohelet set out her arcane equipment, which looked both surgical and culinary. The adult women, more familiar with blood and cooking, were matter-of-fact and stalwart.

This was the same mohelet–a handsome woman in a nubbly pink suit–who had circumcised Erez twenty-two months earlier. With the air of someone used to explaining herself, she politely brushed aside nervous queries about her authority: "Did you know," she countered, "that females performed the rite in ancient Israel?" As a woman and a convert to Judaism (not to mention a plastic surgeon) she had clearer ideas about her role than did run-of-the-mill mohels, most of whom had inherited their ancient sideline unthinkingly, as others inherit a dental practice. Few would even perform a bris on a child born of Catholic parents, let alone a child adopted by a gay man to be raised with his boyfriend. But this one did so happily, recognizing perforce an idea of Judaism that is more inclusive than the one formulated by medieval rabbis. Indeed, in her mimeographed script for the service, she had slightly doctored the traditional prayers so as to include among the litany of patriarchs the names of suppressed matriarchs as well. Perhaps this was only fitting, since the mother had been suppressed in our story, too. Still, in the manner of all things defensive and politically correct, it was as awkward as it was moving: Sarah, Rebekah, Leah, and Rachel had been pieced into the Hebrew text by hand, unevenly, like a ransom note.

There was nothing politically correct about what followed. Onto her forehead, the mohelet strapped a lamp, which glowed and shimmered like a halogen diadem. Then she withdrew from her satchel a large flat board fitted with Velcro restraints. Calmly she instructed me how to hold the baby utterly still upon the board, lest his legs close and ruin the job. In the event, this took all my strength, for he struggled mightily–not, it seemed, from any pain, but from the insult of being butterflied. After saying a prayer, the mohelet dipped the edge of a napkin into a glass of sweet red wine, twisted it into the shape of a nipple and offered it as a mild anesthetic–to the baby, that is, though I could have used it. While he sucked hungrily, she leaned forward and completed the cutting, at which point the baby pooped and promptly fell asleep.

"Our God and God of our mothers and fathers," the mohelet chanted, having added the mothers, "sustain this child and let him be known in the house of Israel as . . . "

Here the script offered only a blank, as life did, too. Andy had wanted to name the child Juan, a nod to his mother, Janet and to the boy's Mexican origins. Zev and Wolf, rejected for Erez, poked up their feral heads again, only to be heartlessly quashed. "You're overcompensating," I told Andy. I suggested honoring his mother with her maiden name–Emanuel–instead; if this were the boy's middle name it would leave us free to choose something pretty and preferably nonanimal for the first. Andy agreed, in part because he liked my suggestion–Lucas, for light–and in part because he thought it sounded ever so slightly like a name that might still mean "wolf."

" . . . let him be known in the house of Israel as Lucas Emanuel," the mohelet continued. "May he bring much joy to his parents in the months and years to come."

With that and a few more prayers, Lucas was a proper Jew, if not to the Orthodox at least to us. But what did that mean: a proper Jew? I was too weak to consider–and oddly famished. I knelt beside my mother's chair and burst out crying. She patted my head, as she always had; my father offered to get me some food from the deli spread Andy had ordered.

"Where do you think it went?" asked my mother a moment later. "You know: *it*. I saw her put it in a napkin, then suddenly it was gone."

"Oh my God," I said, scanning the room for Chauncey.

The Circle of Liberation:
A Book Review Essay of Jesse Green's
The Velveteen Father:
An Unexpected Journey to Parenthood

Jack Drescher, MD

SUMMARY. This essay, in reviewing Jesse Green's *The Velveteen Father*, reflects upon some of the social changes that have surrounded the movement for gay and lesbian civil rights. Prior to the Stonewall riots, postwar homophile organizations like the Mattachine Society affirmed a deep loyalty to the mores of society. After Stonewall, all that changed and accommodationism was out. Post-Stonewall gay liberationists argued that gay men and lesbians would not get their rights by trying to act like heterosexuals. Tragically, the liberatory sexual philosophy of the 1970s could not have envisioned the devastation to be wrought by the AIDS epidemic of the '80s. The gay liberation politics of the '70s would find itself supplanted by other ideologies, such as a call for gay political conservatism or the integration of one's gay identity with traditional religious values. Gay and lesbian politics of the late '80s and '90s, like that of the '50s and early '60s, was to be about fitting into the mainstream. Contemporary discussions surrounding gay and lesbian parenting is a conversation which is not only about a civil rights struggle by gays and lesbians to extract concessions from the heterosexual majority; it also is a conversation within the gay community itself about how one should define a gay identity. *[Article copies available for a fee from The Haworth Document Delivery Service: 1-800-342-9678. E-mail address: <getinfo@haworthpressinc.com> Website: <http://www.HaworthPress.com> © 2001 by The Haworth Press, Inc. All rights reserved.]*

Dr. Jack Drescher is Supervising Analyst, William Alanson White Psychoanalytic Institute, Editor-in-Chief of the *Journal of Gay & Lesbian Psychotherapy*, and author of *Psychoanalytic Therapy and the Gay Man* (1998, The Analytic Press).

[Haworth co-indexing entry note]: "The Circle of Liberation: A Book Review Essay of Jesse Green's *The Velveteen Father: An Unexpected Journey to Parenthood*." Drescher, Jack. Co-published simultaneously in *Journal of Gay & Lesbian Psychotherapy* (The Haworth Medical Press, an imprint of The Haworth Press, Inc.) Vol. 4, No. 3/4, 2001, pp. 119-131; and: *Gay and Lesbian Parenting* (ed: Deborah F. Glazer, and Jack Drescher) The Haworth Medical Press, an imprint of The Haworth Press, Inc., 2001, pp. 119-131. Single or multiple copies of this article are available from The Haworth Document Delivery Service [1-800-342-9678, 9:00 a.m. - 5:00 p.m. (EST). E-mail address: getinfo@haworthpressinc.com].

KEYWORDS. Child-rearing, fertility, gay and lesbian identity, gay liberation movement, gay and lesbian parenting, homosexuality, Stonewall

I am of that generation of men and women who came of age during
the early years of gay and lesbian liberation following the 1969 Stonewall riots. Coming as it did at the tail end of the sixties, the politics of
that movement grew out of a social and political environment that was
anti-establishment, anti-military, and anti-institutional:

> As the sixties came to a close, the United States was a notably
> different country from what it had been a mere decade before . . .
> [when] left-wing agitation no longer marked the national scene,
> and the country remained secure in its self-image as the reposito-
> ry of Rectitude . . . By the close of the sixties, that smugness had
> come undone. Within a six-month period from late 1967 to early
> 1968, the maverick Eugene McCarthy announced for the pres-
> idency; the Tet offensive in Vietnam blew apart the claims of an
> inevitable American victory; the police in Orangeburg, South
> Carolina, fired on black demonstrators, killing three and wound-
> ing dozens; Martin Luther King, Jr., was assassinated, and en-
> raged black Americans rioted in dozens of cities; college students
> across the country took over campus buildings to protest war-re-
> lated research; and the assassination of Robert Kennedy seemed
> to many to spell the end of hope for peaceful domestic reform.
> [Duberman, 1994, p. 169]

The social unrest of the time provided its fair share of metaphors for
the burgeoning gay liberation movement, a movement which had
strongly identified itself with what was then known as the politics of
the left. Gay liberation was seen as a metaphoric equivalent of other
forms of liberation: third world countries were to be liberated from
colonial oppression; African-Americans were to be liberated from
white oppression; women were to be liberated from male domination;
gays and lesbians were to be freed from heterosexual oppression.[1]
Freedom from heterosexual oppression meant freedom from con-
ventional, heterosexual beliefs about what constituted acceptable
forms of sexuality. In what would later come to be regarded as the
pre-AIDS era, many gay writers commonly preached in favor of a gay
sexuality which was either subversive or revolutionary. Consider, for

example, John Rechy's testament to anonymous cruising in *The Sexual Outlaw:*

> The promiscuous homosexual is a sexual revolutionary. Each moment of his outlaw existence he confronts repressive laws, repressive "morality." Parks, alleys, subways, tunnels, garages, streets–these are his battlefields. To the sexhunt he brings a sense of choreography, ritual and mystery–sex cruising, with an electrified instinct that sends and receives messages of orgy at any moment, any place. . . . What creates the sexual outlaw? Rage. [1977, p. 28]

Rechy's call to guerrilla warfare was part of a larger cry for increased freedom of sexual expression, regardless of how much it discomfited the heterosexual majority. Prior to the Stonewall riots, postwar homophile organizations like the Mattachine Society were much more accommodationist in their approach:

> Rather than challenge American values, Mattachine affirmed a deep loyalty to the mores of society. Its goals were fully "compatible with recognized institutions of a moral and civilized society with respect for the sanctity of home, church and state." As if to underline this commitment Mattachine expressly opposed "indecent public behavior and particularly excoriates those who would contribute to the delinquency of minors and those who attempt to use force or violence upon any other persons whatsoever." Finally, while rejecting any affiliation with political movements and parties the Society explicitly declared its commitment to Americanism, avowing a strong anticommunist posture. In the context of the McCarthyite purges of suspected homosexuals, such a stance was hardly surprising from a group that sought to project an image of social conservatism. [Bayer, 1981, p. 71]

After Stonewall, all that changed and accommodationism was out. Just as some African-Americans had earlier argued that it was undignified to straighten their hair or otherwise emulate white people (X, 1964), post-Stonewall gay liberationists argued that gay men and lesbians would not get their rights by trying to act like heterosexuals. Just as black would become beautiful, the overtly sexual gay man would no longer be just a denigrated, heterosexual stereotype; instead he would wear his sexuality as a gay badge of honor (Rotello, 1997). This became one of the defining moments of an era in which calling some-one "promiscuous," was understood to signify envy of their sexual prowess. It was an unbuttoned world in which Kantrowitz (1977) described what he experienced as the stripped-down, utopian egalitari-anism of the gay bathhouse:

> Everything was perfectly blatant. There was no need for shame; we were all wrapped up in similar towels, all seeking our own personal versions of the same thing . . . In our towels we could be sleeping with anyone, a garbageman or an astronaut, and never know the difference. [pp. 184-185]

Tragically, the liberatory sexual philosophy of the 1970s could not have envisioned the devastation to be wrought by the AIDS epidemic of the '80s. And, ironically, the bottle-throwing drag queens at the Stonewall Inn could hardly have imagined that thirty years after their now-famous uprising, the ever-burgeoning movement for gay and lesbian civil rights would be fiercely fought around such establish-ment issues as the delivery of adequate health care (Shilts, 1987), the right to serve in the military (Shilts, 1993; Shawver, 1995), the right to get married (Eskridge, 1996; Sullivan, 1997), and the right to bear, adopt, and/or care for children (Martin, 1993; Green, 1999; Group for the Advancement of Psychiatry, 2000).

It is not difficult to see how this transformation occurred. For many gay people, the call for sexual liberation seemed difficult to reconcile with the call for sexual caution required by the AIDS epidemic (Rotel-lo, 1997). The gay liberation politics of the '70s would find itself supplanted by other ideologies, such as a call for gay political conser-vatism (Bawer, 1993; Sullivan, 1995) or the integration of one's gay identity with traditional religious values (McNeil, 1993; White, 1994; Gomes, 1996). In retrospect, the revolution had succeeded in ways that its early firebrands had never imagined. Although it did not bring about the radical rethinking of acceptable forms of open sexual ex-pression among the heterosexual majority, the liberation movement did sow the seeds of a gay consciousness among subsequent genera-tions. Inevitably, those men and women then shaped the meaning of being gay or lesbian to suit their own generational needs, and then took those identities back to the future: Gay and lesbian politics of the late '80s and '90s, like that of the '50s and early '60s, was to be about fitting into the mainstream. Instead of in-your-face radicalism, gay men and lesbians were once again going to politely ask for a place at the table. As the country's political mood swerved to the right, positions began to emerge which rejected the left-wing politics of earlier gay activists:

> But being gay is not a political act. Homosexuality is not a movement . . . To suggest otherwise is to do none of us any good, and all of us much harm . . . In linking homosexuality with radical politics, [lesbian activist Donna] Minkowitz does not serve the cause of gay rights. Quite the contrary, she is using the cause of gay rights to advance her own program, which would seem to have very little to do with furthering understanding and acceptance of homosexuality as it really exists in America and everything to do with promoting radical-left political ideas . . . [Bawer, 1993, pp. 178-179]

As gay men and women increasingly began coming out into the mainstream of American life, their appearance inevitably led to the contemporary discussions surrounding gay and lesbian parenting. It is a conversation which is not only about the civil rights struggle by gays and lesbians to extract concessions from the heterosexual majority; it also is a conversation within the gay community itself about how one should define a gay identity. After all, the early liberatory equations of the movement did not particularly concern themselves with the raising of children. On the contrary, liberation politics found itself aligned with a growing ecology movement concerned about an overpopulated world. Seen from this perspective, heterosexuals were denigratingly referred to as breeders who conspicuously consumed limited resources. Homosexuality, on the other hand, was not only sterile, it could also be considered environment-friendly.

Yet somehow, some way, the ideology of family values has prevailed. Just as early gay writers put their literary energies into exalting their revolutionary sexplay, some of today's most articulate gay writers have become doting, middle-class parents who are writing about the children they are rearing:

> Lucas (often called Luke or Lukie) was basically a placid baby; when he teethed we hardly knew it. He didn't get frightened, wasn't moody, liked people but was perfectly happy to entertain himself for long periods of time with just a few toys. The outlines of his personality were all there the day he arrived, but now life

was coloring them in–just as it was completing the painting of his physical being, so sketchy once in its prematurity. His Mohawk turned into a shiny, jet-black Beatles shag; his face opened up to the world like a pale magnolia. His eyes became merry. [Green, 1999, p. 194]

Rechy to Green. I'm certain this is not what Kuhn (1972) had in mind when he wrote about paradigm shifts. Having undergone a significant amount of personal psychoanalysis, I am not one to rail against the inevitability of cultural change; nor do I usually find myself longing for a return to imaginary, good old days. Nevertheless, cultural change can sometimes be breathlessly disorienting, particularly for this childless, middle-aged gay man who had watched many of his heterosexual friends disappear into their child-rearing caves/niches during my 20s and 30s. Suddenly, and rather dramatically, I began to see a similar thing happen to gay and lesbian friends after reaching my 40s. Truthfully, I was not entirely prepared or comfortable with this cultural change. When I learned, not too long ago, that the Chelsea apartment above mine had been bought by a gay male couple and that they had just adopted a two-year-old child, this itinerant New York apartment-dweller unexpectedly found himself nostalgically longing for the days when living in a gay neighborhood meant that you didn't have to put up with the noise of young children living in the apartment above.

Having said that, I am loathe to leave the reader with the impression that I am just a curmudgeon in the W.C. Fields mold. As a teenager, I regularly offered to baby-sit for my younger cousins, free of charge. I have always liked, and still like, other people's kids, and some friends' children now call me "uncle." In fact, I am a doting uncle who carries wallet photos of my brother's four progeny, ages 5 to 14 (including twins). Despite the fact that my nephews and niece live in another state, I try to regularly fulfill my avuncular obligations. In fact, at the start of the modern gay liberation movement, being an uncle or an aunt was the only significant child-rearing role envisioned for gay men and lesbians. This did not seem like such a terrible part to play at the time, particularly since it meant that one could be gay and still remain an integral member of one's family. So appealing was this prospect in the '70s, that for those who found comfort in such matters, sociobiologists had even worked out a scientific theory to link a normative view of homosexuality with avuncular, rather than paternal or maternal instincts:

> The homosexual members of primitive societies may have functioned as helpers, either while hunting in company with other men or in domestic occupations at the dwelling sites. Freed from the special obligations of parental duties, they could have operated with special efficiency in assisting close relatives. Genes favoring homosexuality could then be sustained at a high equilibrium by kin selection alone. It remains to be said that if such genes really exist they are almost certainly incomplete in penetrance and variable in expressivity, meaning that which bears of the genes develop the behavioral trait and to what degree depends on the presence of modifier genes and the influence of the environment. [Wilson, 1975, p. 555]

Today's postmodern sensibility tend to make one uncomfortably leery of a scientific narrative which liken the feelings and behaviors of unmarried aunts and uncles to the reproductive habits of bees and wasps. Yet, there is nevertheless something appealing about the theory of kin selection. When my brother and sister-in-law asked me to be their children's guardian, should some unforseeable event prevent them from completing their parental duties, I was honored to be selected as their runner-up. Of course, this contestant wants Mr. and Mrs. America to wear the crown for their entire tour of duty. However, in the event of a tragedy, where and how would I fit children into my already complicated life? Furthermore, can avuncular instincts be transformed into parental ones?

These are some of the questions and issues with which Jesse Green, author of *The Velveteen Father*, struggles, both implicitly and explicitly, throughout this well written, and often moving book. It is written in four sections (see accompanying excerpts in this volume). In brief summary, Green begins with an account of the story of his lover, Andy, in which he chronicles the latter's determined quest to obtain and rear a child of his own. In part two, Green recounts the story of his own childhood and his coming of age as a gay man. In part three, Green meets Andy and his son Erez and, to the author's surprise, their lives intertwine and intersect around the care of the child. Finally, in the last section of the book, they eventually adopt another boy, Lucas.

Green is an able chronicler of this brave new world of gay and lesbian parenting. Until recently, the children of gay people in my generation, and the generations before mine, were usually the results of dissolved heterosexual marriages. "I was married and had kids before I came out," was a phrase often proffered as a paradoxically embarrassed explanation regarding the otherwise proudly-displayed photographs of teenagers, adult children, and grandchildren. Children and grandchildren were sometimes regarded as a strangely, uncomfortable reminder of the days when gay men and women were either in the closet or before they had a conscious awareness of their lesbian or gay identity. Green himself experienced the early categories of the gay liberation movement as quite rigid in comparison to today's gender-bending standards:

> At sixteen, I was pretty much indifferent to babies, never having spent time with them. I didn't fret much about becoming a parent. *Someday, I believed, I would be forced to ask whether I wanted children or wanted to be gay,* but I had a healthy sense that such questions lay far in the future. For now it was enough to wonder if I would ever have sex–and, more important, at which Ivy League college? [Green, 1999, p. 92, emphasis added]

There it was: One had to choose between having children and being gay. One striking parallel with the women's movement should not be lost here: There was a time when a womanly identity meant having to choose between raising children or pursuing a career. Choosing a career was unwomanly (Friedan, 1963). Today women *qua* women struggle with other choices, like how to balance raising a family with a career. Similarly, gay identities have proven to vary according to time, place, and culture. Herdt and Boxer (1993), for example, describe a cohort system of four historical age-groupings of gay men: (1) Those who came of age after World War I; (2) Those who came of age during and after World War II; (3) Those who came of age after Stonewall and the period of gay activism around it; and (4) Those who came of age in the era of AIDS.

The Velveteen Father details some of Green's own losses to AIDS, and he suggests that the HIV epidemic was a major force driving today's "gayby boom." Having children, after all, can be a bittersweet experience. Labor pains precede a birth. The eagerly awaited adoption of a child begins with the tragedy of a mother having to give her child away. Freud (1917) said that the ego is the sum of abandoned object cathexes by which he meant that our perception of reality is frequently shaped by our painful losses. Yet the psychological need to replace the loss of friends and lovers is only part of the AIDS story. Green also notes that the shift toward gay adoption was fueled by an increasingly overwhelmed foster care system that increasingly became swamped with AIDS and crack babies. Ironically, Green, years before he was considering being a parent himself, had written an article that chronicled a NYC agency's first legal placement of a baby with AIDS with two gay men. As he points out, however, gay men are often suspect for harboring parental desires:

> As a source of passion–the kind of passion mothers are admired for possessing and vilified for lacking–fatherhood, even biological fatherhood, was suspicious. Women needed to have children to be seen as normal and fulfilled, but too much child-lust in a man made him a freak: a possible pedophile, or at least homosexual . . . A man who wants to adopt a child is often seen [as] stealing from a woman the one thing society allows (indeed forces) her to keep for herself. Was it finally unnatural–that is, unhealthy–for a man to raise a child without a woman? Was it *selfish?* [p. 22]

The Velveteen Father succeeds in taking the reader on a literate foray into a world in which gay men and lesbians are trying to have and rear children. Essentializing cultural stereotypes would have us believe that lesbians want to have children because they are primarily women, and that they subsequently have an irrepressible maternal instinct. In a similar vein, a heterosexual couple's desire for children is naturalized while the desires of gay men are more difficult to ascertain:

> Ask the parents in a traditional family why they bothered to reproduce and you will most likely get the tautological imperative ("We always wanted to") or a confused collection of rusty saws ("We felt we should give something back to the next generation"). Ask a gay man why he might want to have a child and you're likely to get an uncomprehending stare. For it cannot be overstated how ham-handedly American culture pushes parenthood on heterosexuals and how stingily it withholds the idea from gay men, like an unscrupulous

mountebank. Are you unable to afford a meal, let alone a child? Good, have a baby. Are you fourteen years old and illiterate? Good, have a baby. Are you miserable in your marriage? Good, have a baby. Are you mature and well off and responsible but gay? Good, collect Roseville. [p. 32]

In its chronicle of efforts to overcome biological obstacles to same-sex reproduction, *The Velveteen Father* is a story about relationships, what might be called fertility love affairs; how they work and how they flounder. For example, we learn that before adopting his first child, Andy donated sperm to two lesbian friends, referred to as the two Karens, who were also trying to have a baby. At that time, Andy wanted his own biological child so badly, that he proceeded to participate in making one of them pregnant, despite the fact that his then-lover, Eliot, didn't even like the two women. Eventually, and after several unsuccessful attempts at *in vitro* fertilization, the two women decided to dump Andy for another donor. Although such stories could be easily treated as soap operas, Green eloquently captures the pathos in these affairs:

> . . . the geometry of the lesbian couple at two points of the triangle with the lone sperm donor at the third enforced certain inequities. The inequities were at base biological, of course. The one thing a man lacked in order to give birth to a child was so vast and mysterious that religions were built around it; a woman lacked only a teaspoonful of something men wasted by the gallon. This gave the whole production an unsavory black widow–meets–D. H. Lawrence odor: Come and then die. The putatively virile man so central to the process was actually in the women's employ: a hired hand, as it were. [p. 20]

As a purely narrative account of the personalities and event leading up to an adoption, *The Velveteen Father* is extremely well-written, funny and poignant. Green is a very good writer who made me cry in several places. His story of the crybaby, reprinted elsewhere in this volume, makes a point about the value of tears. In other words, it is a literate book worth reading. However, this book also functions at another level, the mainstreaming political approach of the '90s, and I guess what are now to be called the '00s. This book succeeds at putting a very human face on the lives, desires, and needs of gay men and women. In fact, sometimes it seems as if the audience to whom

Green is often speaking are heterosexual readers who need to be convinced that gay people have feelings too. Since some sections of the book were adapted from earlier articles that were written for mainstream magazines, this perspective is somewhat understandable. However, it can sometimes come across as an unnecessary apologia.

Throughout the book, the reader is struck many times by the fact that sober citizens like Green and his lover Andy can be denied formal legal status to raise their kids as a couple. I found this somewhat unsettling to think about. Yet I remain hopeful as I thought of the many gay men and women who are today raising children. One day these children will grow up. I would like to think that those gay and lesbian parents are in the process of creating a new generation of adults, heterosexual and gay, who will make the world safer for all of us.

The Velveteen Rabbit (Williams, 1922) is an old children's story about a toy rabbit that, through the love of a child, found itself transformed into a real one. In *The Velveteen Father*, the adoptive parent, in this case the oxymoronic gay father, analogously, feels that he becomes "real" through the transformative love of a child. The analyst in me has to wonder if Green means "real" in the sense of Winnicott's (1960) "true self," or of Sullivan's (1953) "authentic" self; the postmodernist in me wants to know, "What is real?"

I do not doubt that a child's love can make some gay people feel real, although I can't help but think that raising children is also what was supposed to make women feel "real" in the 1950s (Friedan, 1963). Certainly, the women's movement has matured, and its mainstream organizations embrace both a women's decision to work outside the home or to stay home and raise kids. For the record, and as seen in one of the sections of the book excerpted in this volume, Green ably documents that child-rearing is also a lot of work.

Perhaps, upon reflection, it is not children, but the possibility of having more options than one had ever imagined that can make a person feel real. In different ways, some individuals strive toward the acquisition of the forbidden, and in doing so they may find different ways to feel real. These forbidden activities could include the right of 1950s women to enter the job market and do "real work," or Rechy's pre-AIDS desire for unrestricted, outlaw sex, or the post-AIDS barebacker's desire for "real sex." If today's quest to be a "real" parent falls in a similar category, two gay men struggling with baby bottles and diaper bags may also be engaged in a revolutionary act. Forbidden fruit indeed.

NOTE

1. It should be noted, however, that many on the political left did not very much care for the gay liberationists' appropriation of their own liberatory metaphors and they often refused to equate the struggle for gay and lesbian rights with those of their own movements.

REFERENCES

Bawer, B. (1993), *A Place at the Table: The Gay Individual in American Society.* New York: Poseidon Press.

Bayer, R. (1981), *Homosexuality and American Psychiatry; The Politics of Diagnosis.* New York: Basic Books.

Duberman, M. (1994), *Stonewall.* New York: Plume.

Eskridge, W. (1996), *The Case for Same-Sex Marriage: From Sexual Liberty to Civilized Commitment.* New York: The Free Press.

Freud, S. (1917), Mourning and melancholia. *Standard Edition,* 14:243-258. London: Hogarth Press, 1957.

Friedan, B. (1963), *The Feminine Mystique.* New York: Laurel.

Gomes, P. J. (1996). *The Good Book: Reading the Bible with Mind and Heart.* New York: Avon.

Green, J. (1999), *The Velveteen Father: An Unexpected Journey to Parenthood.* New York: Villard.

Group for the Advancement of Psychiatry (2000), *Homosexuality and the Mental Health Professions: The Impact of Bias.* Hillsdale, NJ: The Analytic Press.

Herdt, G. & Boxer, A. (1993), *Children of Horizons: How Gay and Lesbian Teens are Leading a New Way Out of the Closet.* Boston, MA: Beacon Press.

Kantrowitz, A. (1977), *Under the Rainbow: Growing Up Gay.* New York: William Morrow and Company, Inc.

Kuhn, T. (1972), *The Structure of Scientific Revolutions.* Second Edition, Chicago, IL: The University of Chicago Press.

Martin, A. (1993), *The Gay and Lesbian Parenting Handbook: Creating and Raising Our Families.* New York: HarperCollins.

McNeil, J. (1993), *The Church and the Homosexual, Fourth Edition.* Boston, MA: Beacon.

Rechy, J. (1977), *The Sexual Outlaw: A Documentary.* New York: Dell Books.

Rotello, G. (1997), *Sexual Ecology: AIDS and the Destiny of Men.* New York: Dutton.

Shawver, L. (1995), *And the Flag was Still There: Straight People, Gay People and Sexuality in the US Military.* New York: Harrington Park Press.

Shilts, R. (1987), *And The Band Played On.* New York: St. Martin's Press.

Shilts, R. (1993), *Conduct Unbecoming: Gays and Lesbians in the U.S. Military.* New York: St. Martin's Press.

Sullivan, A. (1995), *Virtually Normal: An Argument About Homosexuality.* New York: Knopf.

Sullivan, A., ed. (1997): *Same-Sex Marriage: Pro and Con.* New York: Vintage Books.

White, M. (1994), *Stranger at the Gate: To be Gay and Christian in America.* New York: Simon & Schuster.

Williams, M. (1922), *The Velveteen Rabbit.* New York; Doubleday, 1958. http://www.writepage.com/velvet.htm.

Wilson, E. (1975), *Sociobiology: The New Synthesis.* Cambridge, MA: Belknap Press.

Winnicott, D.W. (1960), Ego Distortion in terms of true and false self. In *The Maturational Processes and the Facilitating Environment.* New York: International Universities Press, 1965, pp. 140-152.

X, Malcolm (1964), *The Autobiography of Malcolm X.* New York: Grove Press.

Four Poems

Debra Weinstein

Blessing

Goddess of the basal body, bless us.
Goddess of the reproductive technology,
bless us with the storage tank of #417
at our bedside. Bless the lovers
whose love yields only love.
Make them a daughter, a son.
Bless them in perpetuity.

Debra Weinstein is the author of *Rodent Angel* (NYU Press, 1996).
"Blessing," "Storage Tank," "The Story of Life," and "Little xx" reprinted from *Rodent Angel*, by permission of New York University Press.

[Haworth co-indexing entry note]: "Four Poems." Weinstein, Debra. Co-published simultaneously in *Journal of Gay & Lesbian Psychotherapy* (The Haworth Medical Press, an imprint of The Haworth Press, Inc.) Vol. 4, No. 3/4, 2001, pp. 133-136; and: *Gay and Lesbian Parenting* (ed: Deborah F. Glazer, and Jack Drescher) The Haworth Medical Press, an imprint of The Haworth Press, Inc., 2001, pp. 133-136.

Storage Tank

You house my children
and my children's children.
You are the ship carrying descendant cargo.

You are shrouded in hazardous vapor
like a myth. You hold the ten prong
hanger dangling matter. The one
called back from eternity.

You have been cast off and delivered–
shipped to an office building,
and retrieved in my bedroom.

I do not know what it is like
to awaken suddenly, carried
in the body of another.

The Story of Life

*

These are the enzymes of the gods.
And this is their piss cup.
This is the dropper stuffed with cotton
that transports me back to matter.
I have made love and know
the principles of desire.
I have been love's chemist
alone in my single stall
measuring the elements
that foretell ovulation.

* *

I saw your face in the electron microscope.
It was the frantic face
of the germ cell seeking life.

I saw my os
in the physician's glass.
It was eternity opening
its door a bit wider.

* * *

I wanted you in the biblical sense
as Deborah wanted Deborah.
I pitched my tent by the ocean,
I sang to the armies.
We brewed coffee and
sat all day in the water.
Then fishes circled me
in zebra stripes.

You held my hand.
Later we loved,
shades down.

Little xx

There are orbs on strand *g*
making you a healthy child.
There are crosses marking
the colony of Cell #7.
They come from the unknown
donor, once Christian,
now nothing. Little xx

I cried when they told me
I had a daughter.

Index

Absent parents
  birth mother, 2
  sperm donor, 2
ACLU's Lesbian and Gay Rights
    Project, standards published
    for child custody disputes in
    same sex relationships, 88
Adoption, 81-87. *See also* Agency
    adoptions; Private placement
    adoptions; Second parent
    adoptions
  agency, explanation of, 81-82
  family formation and, 2,66,76
  by gay parents, foster care system
    and, 127
  issues surrounding, 66
  Jewish ritual circumcision and,
    excerpt from *The Velveteen
    Father* about, 117-118
  legal issues, 14,129
  negative feelings about, 14
  prejudice against, excerpt from *The
    Velveteen Father* concerning,
    110-111
  private placement, 81
  reasons for choosing, 18-19
  rise in lesbian and gay families
    formed by, 76
  second parent adoption and, 77
  standard of review, best interests of
    the child, 81
  tragedy of child who is adopted,
    126-127
  transracial issues and, 66
  types of, 81
  The Velveteen Father as story
    about, 128-129
  who will be adoptive parent, 19
Adoption agencies, increased
    acceptance of lesbians by, 8

Adoption information services, local
    gay and lesbian
    organizations, 83
Adoption resources, visibility of, 64
Adoption statutes, language of, 84-85
Adoptions
  foreign orphaned children,
    Immigration and
    Naturalization Service (INS)
    and, 83
  state goals and, 83
Adoptive parent, couple's relationship
    and, 19
Advanced directives
  for gay and lesbian couples, 75
  legal issues to be aware of, 76
  purpose of, 76
Agency adoptions
  foster child and, 81-82
  foster parents and, 82
  risks of, 83
  state involvement with, 81-82
AI. *See* Alternative insemination (AI)
AIC, alternative insemination method,
    both unrelated donor and
    husband, 77
AID, alternative insemination method,
    donor sperm, 77
AIDS
  losses and, 126-127
  sexual liberation and, 122
AIDS babies, adoption and, 127
AIH, alternative insemination method,
    donor husband, 77
Alabama, disapproved adoptions by
    gay men and lesbians, 84
Alternative insemination (AI)
  excerpt from *The Velveteen Father*
    concerning, 109-110
  family formation and, 76